PREGNANCY: A TESTING TIME

Pete Moore PhD conducted research into neonatal development at University College Hospital, London Medical School, before becoming a freelance writer. He is the author of *Born Too Early*, a book for parents of premature babies, and *Trying for a Baby*, about fertility treatments. He contributes regularly to *New Scientist* and *The Lancet* along with other newspapers and magazines. In 1996 he served on a Commission of Inquiry into Fetal Sentience which looked at the issue of fetal pain, and was the main author of its report.

'For it was you who formed my inward parts;
you knit me together in my mother's womb.
I praise you, for I am fearfully and wonderfully made.'

From Psalm 139

Pregnancy: A Testing Time

SO MANY TESTS, SO MANY CHOICES, AND WHAT IF MY BABY IS NOT HEALTHY?

PETE MOORE

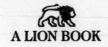

A LION BOOK

Published by
Lion Publishing plc
Sandy Lane West, Oxford, England
ISBN 0 7459 3819 1

First edition 1997
10 9 8 7 6 5 4 3 2 1 0

Acknowledgments
Scripture quotation (Psalm 139) is taken from
the New Revised Standard Version of the Bible,
copyright © 1989 by the Division of Christian
Education of the National Council of the
Churches of Christ in the USA.
William's story on pages 13-16 edited,
with permission, from *Parentwise* magazine

A catalogue record for this book is
available from the British Library

Typeset in 12.25/13 pt Lapidary 333 BT
Printed and bound in Great Britain by
Caledonian International Book Manufacturing, Glasgow

Contents

Foreword

by Caroline Berry

A visit to the antenatal clinic for the mother-to-be of today is a very different experience to the one that her mother would have had. In the 1960s care focused on the mother's health and the only means by which the baby could be investigated before birth was by X-ray. As this technique was known to have a degree of risk it could only be used sparingly.

In 1967 abortion for fetal abnormality had become legal and the stage was set for a huge expansion in fetal testing, occasionally with a view to improved treatment for the fetus or newborn, but more often so that a couple had the option of abortion where serious abnormality was detected.

In the 1970s it became possible to obtain cells for testing from the baby by sampling the fluid that surrounds him or her. This test (amniocentesis) was offered to older mothers and to those with some particular need, usually related to a sad outcome of a previous pregnancy. During this decade ultrasound started to give exciting but blurred pictures of the baby growing silently in the womb.

Tests that involve the baby itself have an inherent risk, so it was only those in special high-risk groups who were likely to be tested then. Other women, who gave birth to an affected child and were offered a test in their next pregnancy, asked wistfully (or angrily) 'why was I not tested last time?'

Further research and the amazing improvements in ultrasound technology have provided an answer to that question, in that it is now possible for any woman to have a variety of tests to obtain information about the developing baby.

But most 'advances' have drawbacks; while a new mother in the 1960s could only ask: 'Is the baby all right?' at the time of birth, today's mother anxiously asks that question on several occasions throughout her pregnancy. Fortunately, for most mothers the answer is reassuring. However, for a small proportion the answer is: 'No!' or, perhaps even more difficult to handle: 'We are not sure; you must come back next week (or later) before we can give you more information.' Suddenly the excitement and joy of being pregnant is replaced by worry and acute anxiety.

During my years of seeing people who were struggling with these difficult situations, I learned that one of the major stresses is the total unexpectedness of a problem result. People have tests to reassure themselves that all is well, and a difficult result often comes as a crushing surprise. It is clear that today's parents need to be aware of today's tests and their implications. I am delighted that Pete Moore has written this book to inform couples and to help them be more prepared for all eventualities. He writes as a Christian but, as the human stories he tells illustrate, this book is an important read for those who have any religious faith, or who have none, because the difficult decisions that may have to be made are equally distressing for all. I am happy to recommend it and hope it will be widely read, lent and discussed.

Caroline Berry MB, BS, PhD, former Clinical Director of the South Thames (East) Genetics Centre, based at Guy's Hospital, London.

1

So you are pregnant

Pregnancy used to be a time of waiting. Now it is a time of assessment and choice.

It may be a surprise, it may be planned, or you may have tried for years, but finding that you are pregnant is a profound moment—often equally for the father—particularly if it is for the first time. Every time I meet a woman who is pregnant, the idea that someone is growing inside her never ceases to amaze me.

Part of the process of coming to terms with the new situation is starting to tell people. You will need to break the news to members of your family, some of whom may be more surprised than others. Friends may laugh, cry or try to ignore your news, but your doctor has to act. One of the first questions he or she is likely to ask with a veiled apology is, 'How do you feel about your pregnancy?' In other words, 'Do you really want to have a baby?' From the outset there is the implication that you still have a choice about whether the child will be born.

In the majority of cases the answer is positive, 'I'm excited, thrilled, daunted but happy...' Others are less sure. Having a baby at this stage in your life could be the very last thing you intended. Or you may be anxious that the child you are carrying could have a serious illness because of your age or because your family has a history of being affected by a specific disease. In some cases, anxiety over the health of the unborn baby may cause you to hold back your emotions and avoid forming any attachment to 'the pregnancy' until tests can show that 'it is healthy'. Unless your decision is to end the pregnancy without further thought, you are more than likely to embark on an impressive battery of tests.

Until remarkably recently the nine months between conception and delivery were veiled in myth and superstition. People used to think that before birth, babies were inert passengers simply awaiting permission to be born so they could start to live. More recent notions that a baby can experience simple forms of learning, hearing and even tasting, would have been laughed out of court.

Many people wish that the closeted world of the unborn child had not been disturbed. Accusations of 'playing God' are levelled at people who probe, however gently, into the womb. Others point out that if we value the life of an unborn baby we ought to give him or her the best healthcare we can provide. For that to occur doctors and scientists need to discover what normal development looks like, and how they can assist individuals who are not following that pattern.

As our knowledge about life in the womb increases, a growing assortment of tests has been developed. Some of them keep an eye on the mother, checking that she remains in good health throughout the pregnancy. These are fairly straightforward and pose few moral or ethical dilemmas. They simply monitor healthy women involved in a normal, natural pregnancy. In fact, so few of these tests ever point to any dangerous development that some people are questioning whether they should be offered at all, or much less frequently.

Another set of tests looks more specifically at the health of the baby, checking for general development and alerting doctors and parents to the possibility that the baby may have a specific abnormality. Here the ethical problems start.

To test, or not to test?

Now that tests are available, everyone is affected. The first choice you are faced with is whether or not to take a particular test. A decision not to have a test is still a decision.

If you go ahead and have the tests, you then have to deal with the results, and that information is seldom straightforward. Many tests simply show the chance the baby has of being affected by a particular condition, rather than a clear cut 'yes, the baby is healthy,' or 'no, there seems to be some problem.' The tests tend to be offered to everyone. Some tests look for conditions that are more likely to occur in babies born to older mothers. These are more strongly recommended when the woman is over 35 or 37 years old; the exact age cut-off depends on your local healthcare policy.

Other tests give a confident statement about whether the baby is going to be affected by some condition. However, some of these have the drawback that they give little or no guidance as to whether the symptoms will be so mild that they will hardly affect day-to-day living, or so gross that a normal lifestyle will be impossible.

There is the real possibility that, as a result of the tests, you may have to make decisions that you will live with for the rest of your life. You may choose to continue with the pregnancy, or you may choose to seek a termination. Either way, you have to choose. It is very hard, probably impossible, to have a test, see the results and then decide to ignore them. You therefore need to be very sure, before having any test, exactly what sort of information it is going to give you, and that you have thought through exactly what actions you may then have to take. If you are beginning to think that this seems like hard work, then you are beginning to understand what is involved.

In her book *The Tentative Pregnancy*, Barbara Katz Rothman argues that the very existence of tests has forever changed the nature of pregnancy. She believes that many women now try not to acknowledge that they are pregnant until after the growing baby has been given a clean bill of health. Lots of couples delay telling anyone about the pregnancy until after the test results are back. In addition, Rothman claims that pressures are placed on pregnant women to conform and have tests so that they don't burden society with extremely needy offspring. This is in danger of turning women into baby-machines controlled by other people's decisions.

If you suggest that any pressure is put on women to take specific tests, the medical community throws up its hands in protest. But healthcare professionals are very aware of their need to protect themselves. In some areas, if a woman declines certain screening tests, the woman has to sign a box in the midwife's notes (the Booking Form) stating that she has been offered the tests, but has chosen to turn them down. This officially is not intended to pressurize the woman, but it makes it clear that she has made a decision that her local health authority is concerned about.

The problem for the health authorities is that they are increasingly being taken to court by parents of babies with diseases that could have been detected by a screening test. The parents argue that if they had had the test they would have aborted the child, so it is the health authority's fault that this child was born. These actions are normally brought so that the parents can win compensation and have the financial resources to provide the additional facilities that their child will need. All of this is extremely expensive for the health authority, so they need written confirmation that you have turned down a test, just in case you try to sue them in the future.

On top of this there is a growing trend towards healthcare professionals having to meet targets of how many people they succeed in getting to take specific tests. At the time of writing this book this trend does not include antenatal screening tests, but it is likely to do so in the near future. If so, it could lead to another source of pressure on couples where the healthcare team has a vested interest in encouraging them to participate. Within this is a desire to reduce the cost of looking after sick people in society. This is fine when it is aimed at reducing the number of people who are sick, but becomes more sinister when it turns into a policy of reducing the number of sick people.

Having a test out of curiosity is not always a good idea. As we will see, a number of the tests carry with them a significant risk of causing a miscarriage. The decision is therefore complicated, as you balance the risk of not knowing about a particular illness or condition, with the risk of inadvertently terminating the pregnancy.

You may feel that the balance swings in favour of testing if you know that a particular illness runs in your family. In this case, screening may bring peace of mind—or it may confirm your fears.

On the other hand, you may feel that the tests are completely unnecessary, as you would not terminate the life of your unborn baby even if tests showed that he or she had a gross abnormality. However, again it is not that simple. One real advantage of having some of the antenatal tests on offer is that specialists can be alerted to any problems before the child is born. This means that they can be ready and able to provide the best level of support immediately after birth, when saving minutes can save a life. Therefore, in some circumstances having the tests can enhance the chance of a sick baby surviving.

A number of couples each year are told that tests show their baby is not at an increased risk of having the particular conditions shown up by that test. Understandably they take this as the reassurance they wanted that their child is definitely healthy. When the baby is born with some abnormality they are extremely shocked. The cause of this discrepancy may be that the test results gave a false impression of health, or that the child is

affected by a disease that was not the subject of any tes
these couples find it harder to come to terms with the
disability than do couples who were never given th
reassurance.

And what are you going to do if a test shows that your baby
has some disability or abnormality? What are the implications for
any children you may already have? Can you afford the extra
costs that are an inevitable part of having a disabled child? Do
you think you could cope?

So, there are implications to both having the tests and not
having them. Think about it *before* you have any test—not after.
A large number of doctors and midwives feel that far too many
people take these tests without seriously considering the
consequences.

My purpose in writing this book is to explain the scientific
basis of all the commonly used tests, and give guidelines on how
to interpret the results. I hope that it will enable you to make
decisions that you are happy to live with.

William

---

*William has Down's syndrome. An antenatal test predicted it. While his
parents have no particular religious convictions, they decided that they
could not have an abortion.*

---

*'Just before Christmas 1994 I received a phone call from the hospital. My
alpha-fetoprotein (AFP) test had come back low—a result which indicated
a higher risk of Down's syndrome. I'd had the test with my previous
pregnancies, always making the same blasé comment that I would rather
know in advance if there was something wrong with my baby. But, as with
all the bad things in life, I didn't think it would happen to me.*

'John and I went to the clinic the next day, expecting to hear that our risk was about 1 in 100. We already knew that, as I was over 30, my risk was at least 1 in 574. However, we were stunned. The doctor considered the risk of our baby having Down's syndrome was 1 in 21. All the questions I'd planned to ask went out of my head as I sat and wept.

'We decided that we couldn't wait until the birth to find out if our baby had Down's syndrome, and booked in for an amniocentesis test. That night I contacted the Down's Syndrome Association and Support Around Termination for Fetal Abnormality. Both organizations sent lots of useful literature. We read everything we could lay our hands on, had the further test, and discussed what would happen if our baby had Down's syndrome. John was very positive that it wasn't a reason to terminate the pregnancy.

'Eight days later, at 5.30 pm, I answered the door to find my GP on the step. His face said it all, but I asked him anyway. "I'm sorry, but your baby has got Down's syndrome." I wept and he hugged me and made small talk with my two small boys, who must have been wondering what on earth was going on.

'I'd never been very optimistic about the result, but having it confirmed was still a dreadful shock. My GP was wonderful, gently questioning me to find out what the next step might be and our reasons. Concerned that John wasn't home, he even offered to stay until he arrived.

'John and I had never felt that we were owed perfect, healthy children. We knew any of us could, through illness or accident, end up with the same as or less potential than this new baby. It didn't seem right to get rid of a baby who was so active. It felt as if he was in there shouting, "Don't forget me; I'm real too!"

'We had a detailed scan a week later. I went with mixed feelings. Part of me wanted to find that our baby was healthy, part almost hoped for catastrophic defects that would take the decision out of our hands. For two days before the scan he had been very quiet. I thought he might be dying. But during the scan he became very active. We discovered we were expecting another son, and whatever other problems he had, he had a sound heart and gut. Having watched him on the scanner for 40 minutes I felt glad he was healthy. We named him William.

'As the pregnancy continued, I became tired of people saying how brave we were, and how loving are children with Down's syndrome. I was perfectly aware that children with Down's syndrome are not genetically "nice" and can still be as difficult—often more so—than another child. I wanted to tell them I already had two loving children, and I didn't need a chromosomal fault to have a loving child.

'I became increasingly depressed. I focused on the negative aspects of Down's syndrome. I wept for my own lost future. I grieved for the child I'd lost—the healthy one who would be like his brothers. I didn't want a child whom people wouldn't be able to understand. I was sad for the child who would learn that he was different, who would be mocked, and who would have to work so much harder for even the simple things that we take for granted.

'I was constantly close to tears, but put on a brave face and told everyone I was all right. John understood, but saw it in a much more clear-cut way—we had done the right thing for our family and we would cope.

'I wasn't coping. I wasn't used to feeling like that. I didn't like it. Eventually, with the encouragement of a friend, I phoned the Down's Syndrome Association, who encouraged me to contact my health visitor. After that it got better—it was still bad, but at least I was able to unload it all at regular intervals.

'Towards the end of my pregnancy, William had hardly moved. I thought this was because his muscle tone was so poor that he would scarcely be able to breathe or feed. Sometimes I thought he must have died, and would be disappointed when he moved. I felt cheated of being able to enjoy my pregnancy.

'William was born on 17 April, four weeks early. He spent a couple of minutes with the paediatrician in the delivery suite, then he was handed over to us. There, after all the fuss and upset, was our beautiful baby boy.

'I still feel glad we knew in advance. The pregnancy was dreadful, but I feel sure that I had worked through the worst of my grief before William arrived. We were able to welcome him into our family with love and knowledge of his special needs.

'William is now one year old. He is a delight, and dearly loved by us all. We have support from our health visitor, a physiotherapist, a home teacher and a speech therapist. He is so much better than we ever expected. It isn't always easy, and we know there will be difficult times ahead—but we all have a future.'

2

The womb is a wonderful world

Before birth a baby follows a clearly identified pattern of physical development, but there is a range of opinions about when a developing baby attains the full status of a human being.

Before we look at the tests themselves, and their consequences, I think it is worthwhile pausing to look at what, or rather who, we are testing. It is also informative to notice the language that different people use in different situations to describe the subject of the tests.

When most women are asked to describe their feelings as they leave an ultrasound scan, they refer to the enjoyment they felt at seeing 'my baby'. Very few use the scientific/technical term of fetus, which for most people conjures up in their mind an alien blob that is far removed from the well-formed child they saw on the screen.

But this is not always the case. On a television debate recently[1] people defending their right to have an abortion referred to their desire to end 'the pregnancy'—i.e. it's my pregnancy, so it's my choice. No mention of the womb's contents at all. Others argued for the use of the word fetus as this acknowledged that something was inside, but was free from excessive emotional overtones. Still others would only refer to the developing individual as a baby, pointing out that if he or she were born after 23 weeks of gestation he or she would be called a premature baby rather than a well-developed fetus, so why not call him or her a baby before birth?

Exploring another world

At conception the embryo consists of a single cell which soon starts to divide. Three days later the embryo is a solid ball of 16 or so cells that, under the microscope, looks rather like a mulberry. Towards the end of the first week the cells are beginning to move to form a fluid-filled space in the middle, with many of the cells collecting together in a main mass. All this usually happens as the embryo travels down the fallopian tube leading from the woman's ovary into her womb.

During the second week of life the embryo implants into the lining of the mother's womb and, from then until birth, will draw nutrients and oxygen directly from the mother's bloodstream. By the end of the third week the embryo has a primitive blood system, and by the end of the eighth week almost every organ is in place. Doctors and scientists now refer to the individual as a fetus rather than an embryo, signifying the completion of development into a recognizable human being.

The past few decades of scientific exploration have led us to realize that before birth a baby acquires a remarkable range of capabilities. By the time a baby is born he or she can move, hear, taste and smell, see, feel, respond to touch and painful stimuli, and learn a few identifying features about his or her mother.

Studying this period of development has made scientists realize just how well the baby is designed for life inside the womb. For years they looked for patterns of behaviour that matched those of infants or adults. Quite often the results of these investigations were confusing. Only recently have they started to look for behaviour and responses that are appropriate to an unborn baby. Now some clarity is appearing in their results.

Movement and responding to touch

Just five and a half weeks after conception, the embryo starts to move. At this stage, movements can be triggered by something brushing against the embryo's lips and over the next two weeks the sensitive area rapidly extends to include the remainder of the face. Three weeks later, touching the palms of the hand will make the unborn baby move and by 14 weeks after conception the whole body is sensitive, with the exception of the back and top of the head.

'A fetus lives in a very different environment from neonates, infants and adults. Consequently, the abilities of the fetus will be tailored to his environment.'[2]

Hearing and memory

Until the late nineteenth century unborn babies were thought to be deaf as well as dumb. This is now realized to be far from the truth. We now think that unborn babies may be able to respond to sound from as early as 12 weeks after conception.

Growing in the womb, an unborn baby lives in a fluid environment. This has a number of important implications. Any sound generated outside the woman's body will be dampened and altered in nature as only lower frequencies will penetrate to the unborn baby. On the other hand, noises produced inside the woman's body—such as the noise of her heartbeat, rumbling tummy, or voice—will carry to the unborn baby very efficiently.

Researchers have found that unborn babies respond to frequencies of between 83 Hz and 5,000 Hz. This is a somewhat narrower range than that of a healthy adult which is considered to be between 30 Hz and 20,000 Hz, with the upper limit dropping to around 8,000 Hz in old age.

Not only can the unborn baby hear noises and make some form of immediate response; there is now strong evidence that an unborn baby learns and remembers certain sounds that are heard frequently. A number of pieces of research point to babies being able to recognize their mothers' voices immediately after birth. The theory is that the unborn baby hears the mother's voice throughout each day. Voices of other people are heard less often and will not be conducted to the unborn baby with anything like the same intensity. They may barely rise above the level of background noise. Another source of evidence has come from babies whose mothers during pregnancy often watched television programmes with clear theme tunes, such as soap operas. After birth, the babies are often pacified by the sound of the theme tune. Both of these examples indicate that some form of learning and memory are possible before birth.

Based on these ideas, many couples like to play music to their babies before they are born, in the hope that this will encourage them to be musical. That is probably stretching things a bit, but it can't do any harm and gives you a way of interacting with your baby during the long wait between conception and birth.

When studying whether an unborn baby could respond to sound, one group of scientists stumbled across the finding that when they exposed unborn babies to repeated stimuli, they responded at first and then ignored it. This sort of behaviour is well known in adults, and is called habituation.

Habituation is an essential screening process that allows us to ignore persistent stimuli, but respond to any new stimuli. For example, if you sit down on a chair you will feel the chair through your bottom for a moment or two. Then you will no longer be able to feel the chair unless you wriggle around a little, or the chair suddenly moves. Signals are still coming from the sensors in your bottom that they are touching a surface, but your central nervous system is choosing to ignore this information. In this way, habituation is one of the simplest forms of learning. These scientists found that, as far as hearing was concerned, habituation was present in human unborn babies from 23 weeks after conception.

Taste and smell

The amniotic fluid surrounding an unborn baby is rich in chemicals. These can be detected by special sense organs in noses and tongues, leaving the possibility that an unborn baby experiences both olfaction and taste. This possibility has been confirmed in a variety of different experiments.

Late in pregnancy a baby will swallow around 500 ml of amniotic fluid a day; a very similar amount of milk will be drunk immediately after birth. In one experiment, doctors injected saccharine into the fluid surrounding the baby. These individuals then started to swallow more fluid than babies living in unaltered fluid. Babies in fluid that was deliberately made to taste sour swallowed less fluid. The take home message appears to be that even unborn babies may have a 'sweet tooth', or should we say a 'sweet gum'!

Before birth, babies also appear to be able to learn about the taste of their mother's diets. Doctors noticed that babies whose mothers normally ate spicy food had more difficulty starting to breast-feed than babies born to mothers who ate more bland diets. When they investigated this further they came to a curious conclusion. The problem seemed to be associated with a change in the mother's diet when she went into hospital to have the baby. Hospital food tends to be non-spicy, so babies who were used to their mothers eating spicy food were expecting to find some of that flavour in her milk. As she was eating hospital food, the flavours were absent and the baby was unwilling to suckle well. Babies whose mothers always ate plainer food did not experience a change and had no difficulty recognizing their mother's milk.

Vision

Not much light gets through a woman's clothes, skin, gut and womb to arrive at the unborn baby. However, doctors believe that the unborn baby is quite capable of detecting light from 26 weeks of pregnancy onwards. It is possible that if a woman in late pregnancy sunbathes in a bikini on a summer's day her unborn baby may see a faint, red glow.

The question of pain

Ten years ago there was no question. As far as experts in fetal development were concerned, before birth a baby was so poorly developed that it could not feel pain. They didn't stop there. Until 1987 there was no scientific evidence that newborn babies could feel pain. The wriggling and screaming that babies showed when an injection was given was thought to be simply a reflex reaction and no emotional response was involved.

Opinion started to change when doctors discovered that if babies were given painkillers during and after an operation, they recovered more rapidly than babies who were merely given drugs that stopped them wriggling. Along with further evidence, this has led to the firm opinion that babies born at term are capable of feeling pain. But what of premature babies?

Neonatal intensive-care units now look after babies that are born after only 23 weeks of pregnancy. Most of the doctors and nurses on the units believe that even these tiny babies are capable of feeling pain, and painkillers are frequently used. So if a 23-week-old premature baby can feel pain, it makes sense to think that a 23-week-old unborn baby can also feel pain if exposed to a painful stimulus like a syringe needle.

Research in this area is scarce, but a team of doctors and scientists at Queen Charlotte's Hospital in London have published results from a number of investigations. These show that during needling procedures the concentration of stress hormones in the baby's blood increases more than sixfold. The unborn baby also sends more blood to his or her brain and reduces the amount going to the rest of his or her body. Both of these responses indicate that the baby has detected the needle and has raised a biological alarm. Whether this is exactly the same as adult pain remains to be answered, but these reactions have been seen in unborn babies after only 15 weeks of pregnancy.

At the time of writing this (early 1997) the newspapers have been full of comments about whether or not an unborn baby can feel pain. Some people are amazed that anyone ever raised the question—of course an unborn baby could feel pain they say. Others are equally certain, but in the opposite direction. For them, you can only feel pain after birth. The rest of us are left in the middle trying to sort it out.

What is clear is that if an unborn baby is injured he or she clearly detects it and mounts a defensive response. But has the baby felt pain?

For the baby to feel pain the part of the brain that controls that ability must be up and running. And this is where the problems start. No one really knows which parts of the brain you need in order to feel pain. Some say that you must have a fully functional cortex, the incredibly complex layer of nerve cells that covers the top of the brain. Others say you can have some rudimentary sensation of pain as soon as an area of the mid-brain called the thalamus is working. Still others say that you can't rule out the possibility of an unborn baby feeling pain as soon as there are some working nerves.

To put some time scales on this, the first nerve cells start to function during the fifth week of growth, the thalamus starts to operate at around 11 weeks and the cortex is functional and connected to the rest of the brain by 24 weeks after conception.

Most doctors and scientists believe that for the moment the jury is out. There is little doubt that an unborn baby has some ability to experience pain once he or she has reached 24 weeks after conception, and that this ability may extend considerably earlier. Consequently the medical community is debating whether they should try to anaesthetize unborn babies before performing invasive treatments. But as we know very little about the long- or short-term effects of standard anaesthetics on unborn babies, it will be some time before this matter is resolved.

Set up for life

It's not just that an unborn baby may feel pain if injured. Scientific experiments have shown that a stimulus given to an unborn baby permanently modifies the connections in the spinal cord. If the stimulus is pain then the nervous system becomes sensitized to pain and for the rest of the person's life they will perceive a small injury as producing a greater amount of pain than would otherwise have been the case. So whether or not the unborn baby 'feels pain' before 26 weeks, there is a growing realization that it is important to minimize an unborn baby's exposure to noxious stimuli so that his long-term neurological development is not perturbed.

This is starting to change the way that newborn, premature infants are treated by doctors during potentially painful procedures. They are now given much more pain relief to block the passage of signals to the spinal cord and prevent these changes taking place.

On top of this, there is now a substantial body of evidence that the nutritional status of a growing unborn baby radically affects his or her susceptibility to particular diseases later in life. In particular, poor prenatal nutrition can leave a person prone to heart disease, stroke, diabetes or high blood pressure. The phenomenon is known as fetal programming.

The theory is that while the genes we inherit are unique, the way they are expressed is influenced by the environment in which the person grows up and lives, including the environment experienced in the womb. The unborn baby will compensate for poor nutrition by making adjustments to the way that he or she is growing, attempting to maintain an adequate nutrient supply to the developing brain at the expense of the rest of the body.

This suggests that a developing baby is therefore highly sensitive to environment, not only in the sense that he or she can feel the environment, but in that the environment in the womb will strongly influence the way the baby develops subsequently. Table 1 shows how quickly the baby develops in the womb.

Is birth 'day one' of life?

'How old are you?' A simple enough question, but one that is normally answered somewhat inaccurately. Normally, the age given is the time that has passed since the person's birth, which has the underlying suggestion that prior to that date he or she didn't exist. Clearly that is not the case.

Within any group of people you will normally find a wide range of responses if you try to probe harder and ask their opinions about when they believe life begins.

Conception

The moment of conception, when sperm and egg combine to form a cell with a unique set of genes, is seen by many people, particularly those holding strong religious convictions, as the moment that a person's life starts. They claim that the desire to date the beginning of life at a later point is driven mainly, or even solely, by a wish to perform some procedure that would be considered unethical on a human being.

The issue is not whether this fertilized cell is capable of performing any particular functions, but that it has the potential of performing all human functions at some point in the future. After all, there is no point at which all of our faculties are functioning perfectly. By the time we are sexually mature we are losing millions of brain cells a day and still learning to be mentally mature. By the time middle-age vigour gives way to old-age wisdom, we are physically less capable. If a person is only human when they are performing to their full potential then we should all give up now.

Others say that it is not quite that simple: this joining of egg and sperm is a process occurring over many hours—it doesn't define a single moment. Also, there are many hurdles to be overcome between conception and birth, with more fertilized eggs failing to develop into babies than succeeding.

Twinning

The growing bundle of cells can split into two and form identical twins at any time over the first few days after fertilization. Therefore, until this period is over you cannot be certain whether one or more 'persons' are going to develop from the fertilized egg. Surely, say some, you need to wait at least until you know how many 'persons' there are before you can say that a life has started.

Weeks of pregnancy	Observation	Crown–rump length*
0	First day of last period	
2	Ovulation	
3	Embryo implants in womb	
5	Arms start to form	3 mm
8	You can start to see movement	16 mm
9	Isolated head, arm and leg movements and hiccups	24 mm
10	Baby has distinctly human appearance and a fully formed heart. Fetal breathing movements can be seen at an ultrasound scan	33 mm
11	CVS (chorionic villus sampling) may be performed	
12	It is possible to identify the sex of the baby, which can be seen sucking and swallowing	75 mm
16	AFP, Bart's test and Leeds test may be performed	
16	Some mothers start to feel occasional movements	125 mm
16	Amniocentesis may be performed	
18–20	Routine ultrasound scan to check the baby's development	
20	Most mothers feel movements by now	180 mm
24	Babies born from now on have a chance of surviving	230 mm
28	The baby opens his eyelids. Most babies born after this age survive	260 mm
36	Fingernails reach the end of the fingertips	300 mm
40	The official due date	340 mm

Table 1: Progress of development and growth of an unborn baby.
*As it is often very difficult to measure the complete length of an unborn baby (i.e. from head to toe) measurements are usually made from the top of the head to the bottom—crown to rump.

Implantation

Other people say that a person's life has started when the embryo is implanted into the womb. This is complete by about 14 days after the egg and sperm have met. They point out that in the normal situation up to 75 per cent of fertilized eggs fail to implant. The argument maintains that they can't all have been little people, lost before they were 14 days old. After successful implantation, the chance of survival increases enormously.

Nervous system

Another possible choice of a developmental stage is six weeks after conception, when the first parts of the nervous system start to operate. The rationale here is that we decide when a person is dead by looking to see if the nervous system is operating, so why can't we use the same criteria for deciding when life starts?

Again, it is not that simple. Doctors look for the death of nerves in strategic areas of the brain to establish brain death in adults. It is only around 12 weeks after conception that any activity starts in these areas and much later before it becomes organized. The nervous system does not simply turn on one day, but instead follows a progressive pattern of development that is not complete until after birth.

Quickening

The first movements that a woman can feel have always been taken as a significant stage in the baby's development. This is called the moment of 'quickening'. Historically, this has been taken as the moment when the baby's soul enters his or her body. From observations using ultrasound scanners, we now know that this is far from the first time the baby moves. It just happens that this is the first occasion that the baby has lashed out with sufficient vigour with a hand or foot for the woman to feel the thump or kick.

Birth

From the moment a newborn baby takes a breath of air, he or she is legally a person. However, although most babies are born 40 weeks after the woman's last menstrual period, 5 in every 100 are born more than a month early and some that are born four months early survive. If birth is used as the marker of the start of a person's life, then these premature infants start their life four months earlier than everyone else.

Postnatal

At the extreme end, there are philosophers who maintain that babies do not become persons in their own right until they can make decisions. For this, they claim you have to wait a number of months after a baby is born.

My opinion

Like many, I find this hard to resolve. Clearly, conception is the process that forms a unique set of genes. The fact that so many embryos fail to implant, or that a few develop into twins, indicates that there are problems associated with calling this newly fertilized egg a person in every sense of the word. However, to call the fertilized egg anything other than human is also blatantly incorrect.

The question must then move to the moral value and rights of this human embryo. There are clearly occasions where the only way out of a tragic situation is to terminate the pregnancy with an abortion in order to safeguard the woman's life. An example of this would be an ectopic pregnancy, where the baby is growing inside the woman's abdominal cavity rather than inside her womb. If left alone, this will lead to the death of both the mother and her baby. There are two ways of looking at this decision to preserve the woman's life at the expense of her unborn baby. Either I am placing a slightly different moral value on the unborn child than I do on the mother, or I am simply acknowledging that there is no way of saving the baby's life and at least this saves the mother. I think it is probably a mixture of the two.

In cases of extreme handicap, all hard and fast guidelines fail. A baby growing without a brain is clearly not going to survive. A decision to terminate this pregnancy would be quite under-standable. However, what then is classified as an extreme handicap? What if the baby has half a brain, or three quarters—where do you draw the line?

I am convinced that legislation would never be able to give a solution to this. It would either be too weak to be useful, or too strong to have compassion, and public opinion would demand that it was withdrawn or changed. However, I still believe that the general principle we should strive to apply is that a developing baby has an extremely high moral value and it is our duty to offer protection wherever possible.

Notes

1. *Kilroy*, 23 October 1996.
2. Professor Peter Hepper, Director of the Fetal Research Centre, Queen's University, Belfast; Hepper, P.G., 'Fetal psychology: an embryonic science' in *Fetal Behaviour—Developmental and perinatal aspects* (Ed. Nijhuis, J., Oxford University Press, 1992).

3

Understanding the results

To understand the results of a test you must first establish whether it is a diagnostic test or a screening test. To understand the results of a genetic test you must establish the exact way that the particular disease is inherited.

Before we look at any antenatal tests we must understand that they all fall into one of two groups. Some give specific answers to specific questions; for example: is the baby a boy or a girl? These are 'diagnostic' tests. Others only indicate whether you are more or less likely than an average member of the population to be affected by whatever the test is attempting to identify. These are 'screening tests' (see Table 2.)

Diagnostic tests

A few tests can give definite yes-no answers to questions about whether or not the baby has a particular condition. Some of them can also show clearly whether the baby is a boy or a girl.

These tests are able to be clear-cut because they are based on scientific analyses that look at the genetic material inside some of the baby's own cells. Over the past few years, scientists have developed tests that take a closer look at the genetic material.

Their quest has been to identify mistakes in one of the 100,000 genes encoded on the chromosomes. Such a mistake indicates that the baby has a particular disease.

There are various methods for getting hold of the baby's cells, of which amniocentesis and chorionic villus sampling (CVS) are the most common. The choice will largely depend on the age of the pregnancy, although it may also be affected by the doctor's individual preference. These are explained in chapter 6.

While these tests are good at diagnosing a disease, they have three drawbacks. First, they tend to be expensive to perform, so cannot be offered on the NHS to the general population. Secondly, they often cannot tell you how severely the baby will be affected by the condition. It may be mild or severe—only time will tell. Thirdly, some of these tests can trigger miscarriages.

Test	Diagnostic	Screening
AFP (alpha-fetoprotein)		✓
Bart's triple test		✓
Bart's quadruple test		✓
CVS (chorionic villus sampling)	✓	
Amniocentesis	✓	sometimes
Ultrasound scan	sometimes	✓

Table 2: Which tests are diagnostic and which are screening?

Screening tests

An increasing sector of modern medicine is concerned with searching for the early signs of disease in people who believe that they are perfectly healthy. Much publicity has been given to the X-ray programmes that look for breast cancer or the smear tests that attempt to identify women with early stages of cervical cancer. Debate ebbs and flows about the benefit or otherwise of having a similar screening campaign trying to identify men with early stages of prostate cancer. All of these programmes come under the broad banner of screening tests.

The word screening has been very deliberately chosen and it comes from an agricultural source. After the harvest a screen (sieve) is used to separate large cereal grains from smaller grass seeds, dust and dirt. The process is called screening, and how well it works depends on the size of the holes in the screen. If the holes are too small then the chance of an individual piece of rubbish falling through the mesh is reduced. Consequently, a lot of rubbish will be collected with the corn. If the holes are too large there is a strong possibility that good corn will fall through onto the waste heap.

Apply these ideas to medical screening and we can soon see why screening tests seldom give a cut and dried, yes or no result. Instead, they normally give a result that says you are a certain percentage more or less likely to be affected by the particular condition than an average member of the population.

A test looks for some identifiable feature that indicates the presence or absence of a particular disease. Very often it measures the amount of a hormone or some other chemical that is present in healthy people but occurs at either elevated or reduced levels in people with the disease. However there is normally a wide range of results in healthy people and again a wide range in those affected by the condition. Things become complicated as the numbers normally overlap (see Figure 1).

So, where do you set the threshold to decide that the deviation from what you would expect, or hope for, is so great that action needs to be taken? If you set a high threshold then chance will dictate that some people with the condition will not be detected. They will incorrectly believe that there is nothing to worry about. This is called a 'false negative' result (see page 12). On the other hand, if you set the level too low then you will suggest to

An ideal screening test would separate people affected by a condition and those completely unaffected into two clearly separate groups. A test result between 1 and 4 means that the person is unaffected by the condition; a result between 5 and 8 shows that they are affected.

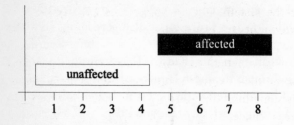

In most screening tests the healthy and unhealthy groups overlap, leading to uncertainty.
A test result of 4 or 5 could mean that the person is either unaffected or affected by the particular condition that this test is assessing.

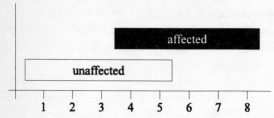

Figure 1: Setting the threshold in screening tests

perfectly healthy people that there might be some problem. Consequently, some who are not at risk will be unnecessarily exposed to anxiety and possibly unnecessary treatment. This is called a 'false positive' result.

Not only do you have problems establishing the threshold levels, but there is also the question of frequency. Do you test every day, just in case something has changed since yesterday, or do you test once and assume that nothing changes? The answer varies depending on the exact test, but it is influenced by the fact that testing too frequently is stressful for the person and expensive for the system. On the other hand, it needs to be sufficiently frequent to catch any ill-health that may be developing.

On top of all this, people who study medical ethics generally agree that it is unethical to give a test that can detect some illness, unless there is something the person can do with the results. In the case of breast cancer screening, early detection of a tumour before it has grown too far allows for the surgical removal of a small area of tissue containing the tumour. The test clearly leads to a worthwhile treatment. However, for many women, the only 'treatment' on offer following the antenatal screening tests is a termination.

The complicating factor with antenatal screening programmes is that even if you are certain you would not abort a child as a result of the test, you and your baby can still benefit from the results. First, they allow you to mentally prepare yourself and your family. Secondly, it allows the hospital to be ready with any additional help your baby may need at birth.

The meaning of 'chance'

So, the test is over and the results are back. Instead of a clear 'Yes' or 'No', you are faced with a 'chance', a 'probability'. It is not possible for the healthcare team to give any definite answer to your question: 'Is my baby affected, or healthy?' They can simply refer to the chance of good health or ill health. That is all the test set out to establish.

It often falls to the unfortunate midwife or health visitor to try and explain probability and chance in relation to testing. What does it mean if the chance of your baby having an abnormality is 1 in 10, or 1 in a 100, or 1 in 100,000?

As a society, we are not helped by institutions such as the National Lottery. Each week the winning numbers flash up on our TV screens and one or two people share the jackpot and become millionaires. For them the 1 in 17 million chance that they picked the correct numbers actually happened. The newspaper photographs of the instant millionaires fuel the feeling that it really could be you next week. When the National Lottery started operating, a rival betting company said that the sort of event they would quote at 17 million to 1 was a light aircraft piloted by Elvis Presley landing on the head of the Loch Ness Monster. My personal opinion is that any nation where a majority of the adult population buy National Lottery tickets in the 1 in 17 million hope of winning the jackpot is not very good at understanding statistics and probability.

Much of our judgment of probabilities is affected by how familiar we are with the situation. The chance of being killed if you travel by plane is vastly lower than the chance of being killed if you travel by car. But it is not unusual for people to make sure that they have made a will before taking their first flight, although they would never have considered the need to do this before getting in a car.

When considering our response to given probabilities, we also weigh up the severity of an adverse outcome. If the problem being predicted is only minor then we will take a greater risk. However, if it is going to be long-term, time-consuming and have the potential of being financially costly, then the tendency to want to reduce the risk becomes greater.

So, one day you move from seeing someone winning when the odds were 1 in 17 million, to finding that a test shows that your baby has a 1 in 200 chance of having a serious abnormality. It is easy to jump to the conclusion that, with a number as small as

The chance of:	Risk:
getting cancer during your life	1 in 3
having asthma	1 in 15
being injured in a UK road accident in any one year	1 in 150
having a stroke at some point in life	1 in 200
developing multiple sclerosis	1 in 1,000
having cystic fibrosis	1 in 2,000
being killed in a UK road accident in any one year	1 in 15,000
being killed in a UK air crash in any one year	1 in 10,000,000
being struck by lightning in any one year	1 in 10,000,000

Table 3: Risks in life

200, this is a high risk and you must do something about it. Table 3 shows some of the risks we face in life.

Let's flick a coin

A brief lesson in statistics is needed, so that people can get their minds around the concept of chance.

Embedded firmly in our minds is the idea that life ought to be fair. We get upset with any indications that this might not be the case. But what do we mean by fair? A couple who already have two boys might feel that it is only fair if the next baby is a girl. They may even feel that because they have had two boys already the chance of getting a third boy if they have another child must be reduced.

A simple game can show where this thinking is wrong. Take a piece of paper and mark on it a grid that has 26 vertical columns and 4 horizontal rows. Label the columns A-Z, representing 26 families. Now these families want to have children and you determine the sex of the child by flicking a coin—heads means the child is a boy, tails means it's a girl (see Table 4).

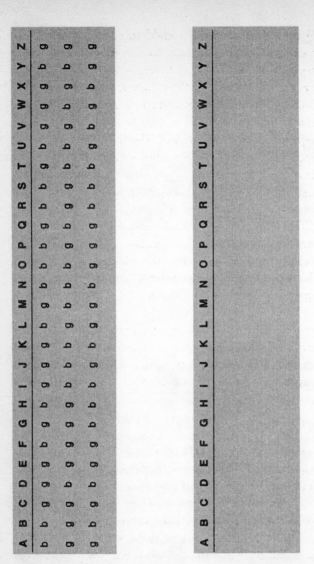

Table 4: Flicking coins. On this occasion I ended up with three all-girl families and one all-boy family. Their parents would easily have expected the third child to ring the changes. However, we can see that the system wasn't biased, as the overall count gave 36 boys and 42 girls, almost half and half.

Go along the first row giving a child to each family. Unless there is something very strange with your coin, you will have a mixture of girls and boys shared between the families. Now repeat this on the second line. By the time you reach the end, you will have some families with a girl and a boy and some with two of the same sex.

Finally, repeat this on the third line. The thing to note now is that the selection of either a girl or a boy as the third sibling to the family is made independently of the first two children.

By the end of this process you will most probably have every combination of family you could imagine, from three girls to three boys. The families with all their offspring of one sex may feel that something odd, maybe even unfair, has happened. But you can check that this is not the case by counting all of the boys and all of the girls. In this large population census, you will find that the numbers of each are very similar.

The thing to note in the whole of this exercise is that at the point where each individual 'person' was created, there was an equal chance that it could be a boy or a girl. This is totally independent of how many boys or girls are already in the family, or, for that matter, of the population at large.

Dealing with a screening result

Your phone rings, or the midwife calls around, giving you the good news that, based on the test results, there is only a 1 in 10,000 chance that your baby has a serious abnormality. Taking your age into consideration, this means that you are substantially less likely to have a problem than the average member of the population. You sigh with relief and make a cup of tea. Sadly though, this is still no guarantee that all is well; all you know is that there is a good chance that everything is fine. It still could just possibly be you.

You may not be so fortunate, and the news may be more

worrying. You may have a 1 in 200 chance of a problem, perhaps even a 1 in 10 chance. The first thing to note is that, in both of these cases, the odds are still in favour of the baby being perfectly healthy. In the first example, out of 200 babies who give this result, 199 will not be affected by the condition and even in the second, 9 out of 10 babies given that screening score will be healthy.

Very often, the expectation is that you will move straight on and have a diagnostic test. You may even feel under a certain amount of pressure to take the tests, but the decision must be yours.

An ultrasound scan is safe, but is often unable to identify any problems even if they exist, so the only options are tests based on a sample of the baby's cells. Here the problem is that the methods used to collect the cells carry some risk of triggering a miscarriage. For amniocentesis, the risk is in the order of 1 in every 200 procedures; for CVS it varies from centre to centre. At centres where the doctors perform a small number of CVS tests each year the miscarriage rate tends to be higher, so always ask to be sent to a large, specialist centre, where the miscarriage rates tend to be 1 in 50 to 1 in 100.

If your test suggests a 1 in 200 chance of the baby having some abnormality, then having an amniocentesis means that it is more likely that the test will cause the miscarriage of a healthy baby than find that the baby is unhealthy. What a choice to be faced with! You may feel at this point that a little information is worse than none, and wish that you had not had the initial test. This highlights the need for couples to consider the consequences of the partial nature of the information they will receive, before agreeing to any tests.

Another thing to remember is that many of the tests apply to conditions that have a wide range of severity. For example, some children with Down's syndrome are severely handicapped, while others are capable of living semi-independent lives as adults.

However, the screening tests are very poor at predicting how severely any individual child will be affected.

Subsequent pregnancies

Understandably, many people who have lost one child because of a severe physical abnormality are deeply worried that it will occur again in a second pregnancy. It appears that in many cases severe abnormalities occur spontaneously in the first few weeks of pregnancy and the actual cause remains a mystery. A post-mortem examination will often give clues about the reason for the malformations, but sometimes the cause will remain unknown.

Just because doctors cannot identify a specific genetic problem does not mean that one did not exist. It is now believed that most malformations have some genetic component, and you would do well to seek the help of a genetic counsellor who will help to determine the risk in your specific situation. As a broad guideline, parents who have had one child with congenital malformations are at a 3 per cent risk of future babies being similarly affected. This is in addition to the 1.5 per cent risk of birth defects that accompany each and every pregnancy.

Chromosomal and genetic abnormalities

This simple rule of chance can be thrown into disarray if there is a specific genetic disease within your family. Genetics is a relatively new area of science, but one that has profound implications. As geneticists have gradually begun to unravel the instructions that give rise to the physical structure of our bodies, they have shed light on the way that many diseases can be passed through families from one generation to the next. Chapter 7 talks in more detail about chromosomal and genetic abnormalities.

Genetic screening and the role of counsellors

Where previously genetic diseases were seen as the realm of mystery, maybe even the judgment of God, we can now identify physical causes. The problem is that the more scientists discover, the more complex the story becomes. Genetic screening tests are becoming available, some by mail order, but the implications of the results for you and your family may not be straightforward.

As we will soon see, the world of genetic disease has some general rules that can help us to understand genetic illness. However, each particular condition has unique features, and each couple who suspect they may be affected need to be given individual expert advice, preferably before they consider trying for a baby.

Enter the genetic counsellors. These people are trained not only to know what tests are available, but also to understand the benefits and limitations that the results will bring. They are also experienced in helping people think through their options and try to grapple with the meaning of the probabilities and chances that they are presented with.

You can see a genetic counsellor by initially going to talk to your General Practitioner (GP). He or she should be able to advise you about whether or not you need to see a genetic counsellor, and arrange an appointment if necessary. If your family background shows clearly that there is a genetic illness present, it is normally best for you to see a counsellor rather than simply discuss the situation with your GP. The waiting times for appointments vary enormously around the country, from a few weeks to many months.

As a couple, your reason for seeking genetic advice may be because one of your children has a severe abnormality and you want to know whether this is due to a genetic condition that one of you is carrying. On the other hand, you may know of a history of disease in members of your family that could have a genetic cause.

A first visit to a genetic specialist may last for a couple of hours. Don't be worried that you can't take in all that you have been told during this session. You should be provided with some written information to read and think about. Further sessions should be booked, so that you can come back with questions. Always try to write your questions down before you come into these meetings, otherwise you are bound to forget some of them at the time.

One of the counsellor's tools is a family tree—your family tree. Early in the discussion, he or she will ask about your relatives and see whether there is any pattern of disease through the family. This information will be needed for the families of both the man and the woman. You need to be aware that in seeking this information you may affect the whole of each family, as before your investigation they could have been completely oblivious to any problem. If you discover that an errant gene is running through one or both families you may be in a position to advise other family members to seek medical advice.

A development to watch for in the future is how insurance companies are going to deal with results from genetic screening. Recently, there have been a few well-publicized cases where this knowledge has suddenly made it impossible for members of the family to get certain insurance policies. However, at the moment the companies are insisting that the vast majority of people will not be affected by anything they discover about their genetic make-up.

Jane

Jane has a PhD and works in the Department of Accounting at a university. Even she found that the way the test results were presented was difficult to cope with. After two sets of tests that disagreed with each other, she gave birth to a healthy baby boy.

'I had a borderline low (whatever that means!) AFP result when I was pregnant for the third time, and was told that the risk of Down's syndrome was about 1 in 270. The doctors recommended amniocentesis. One of the doctors I saw considered I was also in a higher risk for problems because I had miscarried just two months before conceiving this baby.

'I did not want to have amniocentesis, primarily because of the recent miscarriage, so requested a second AFP test. Although they said that their policy was only to offer a second test when the initial result was high, they agreed. Their reasoning is that the AFP level normally increases during this period and a somewhat higher level with retesting would be expected, which would only put me in an even higher risk group. However, since the results are interpreted in the light of how far along the pregnancy is, I reasoned that a retest might provide meaningful information.

'The retest was "normal", indicating a risk of Down's syndrome of about 1 in 780, which was consistent with my age at the time. I also had an ultrasound at this point and the ultrasonographer checked for several characteristics that are common to Down's syndrome babies. She found none. After that, I was able to relax and not worry about the AFP test.

'In the end I gave birth to a healthy baby boy.'

4

Making decisions in a culture of choice

Antenatal tests give the impression that a couple can choose to have a healthy baby. This is an illusion. As a society that values the rights of individuals to make their own choices, we have chosen to provide screening services. In the case of making decisions on behalf of an unborn baby, the law gives the responsibility to the mother.

Before deciding to have any tests, you should consider what you will do with the information you receive. Your decisions will be based on a number of factors, including the status you give to a developing baby, concern about the effects that a child with a disability may have on existing family members and concern for the developing baby.

If screening tests detect some abnormality you will be left with four options (have diagnostic tests, abort, prepare yourself and your family, or, possibly, treat), all of which have long-term implications.

The whole notion of testing introduces the idea that we can control our lives and that we have the authority to take control over the lives of our children. The theory is that if you test for a disease you are in a position to do something about it. A test for breast cancer opens the opportunity of receiving treatment: chemotherapy, radiotherapy, or surgery. You may choose not to have any, but the test gives you the choice; it gives you a measure of control.

When it comes to having babies, antenatal testing is not unique in offering the possibility of some control. Contraception has given many couples the ability to plan when their children come along so that they fit conveniently into their careers. As a result, they can take control over their lives. However, some have found that their control is not absolute as their contraception fails, or conversely they find that, try as they might, they remain child-free.

The reality is that you can have some influence, but you are not in control. You may be able to limit certain risks or solve certain problems, but you can never guarantee good health.

There is nothing to prevent you having all the screening and diagnostic tests currently available for monitoring your baby and still having a child who is born with some severe abnormality. The tests only cover a limited range of conditions. Similarly, no screening test will ever be able to prevent your child suffering an accident and becoming permanently disabled. The accident may occur during birth, when the child is one year old, running around the school playground, or much later in life. The cold reality is that you are not in control—trying to pretend that you are is likely to be a poor way to prepare you for the perils of being a parent.

Rights and responsibilities

The end of the twentieth century has seen 'rights campaigns' flourish. For example, incorporating the values highlighted by women's rights campaigns has led to massive changes in our social structure, and animal rights campaigns have brought about widespread changes in agriculture and laboratory research. On a smaller scale, everyone is now used to calling for their individual rights.

Among these are calls for the right to use any antenatal screening method and follow up with an abortion if the test result is deemed to be unfavourable. Because women carry the babies through pregnancy and are very often the primary carers for children once they are born, the whole area comes under the remit of women's rights. Any argument that would restrict access to these tests rapidly comes up against the formidable strength of the women's movement.

This is an issue because quite often the only 'medical' option on offer after an unfavourable test result is an abortion. Thus, in claiming her right to an abortion a woman has to deny that an unborn baby has an absolute right to life.

In reality, couples are caught in a dilemma of balancing different people's rights. There is the woman, the developing baby, the father and any other children. All have grounds for claiming their rights and all will be affected by the birth of a baby who has some disability.

And what of a couple who find that their unborn baby has an extreme abnormality, such as the absence of kidneys or a brain. In all of these cases the child will die at birth, or shortly after. Is their duty of care so strong that they would be wrong to abort the pregnancy? Does this baby have a right to at least nine months of life in the womb? Under UK law, apparently not. Up to the 24th week of pregnancy, an abortion can be granted for a wide range of reasons. These include the statement that continuing the pregnancy poses a risk, greater than if the pregnancy were terminated, of injury to the physical or mental health of the pregnant woman; or of injury to the physical or mental health of any existing child(ren), or the family of the pregnant woman—the so-called 'social reasons' for abortion. Thereafter, terminating a pregnancy is permissible up until term if the child has a severe malformation—but sadly (or inevitably) there is no definition of what constitutes a severe abnormality.

Pregnant women should be given maximum information, orally and in writing, and made aware that screening is an option and not an obligation. [1]

The rights of existing children must not be forgotten. Having a severely handicapped brother or sister is going to affect the amount of attention they can receive from their parents. It will influence every aspect of home life, from the house you live in to the holidays you take. Many families have found that the children have learned from the experience of caring for a disabled sibling. Other couples have not stood the strain, and their marriages have ended in divorce.

Some people argue that it is unfair to knowingly bring a child into the world who will have a life of pain and distress. The argument is that the baby's right to our care can allow us to prevent this sort of discomfort by preventing the birth in the first place. This is commonly used in debates about whether or not a baby with Down's syndrome should be aborted. It is seen as a sad but necessary act of mercy. Other people argue that the baby has a fundamental right to life, whatever the 'quality' of that life. For example, the Prolife Alliance, campaigning in the 1997 UK general election, said: 'Absolute respect for innocent human life from fertilization until natural death is the keystone of justice. The right to life is the right from which all others flow.'

Balancing the rights of everyone involved in these situations is a dilemma that will never be solved. However, this does not give us a licence to bury our heads and pretend the problem does not exist.

Who decides?

The medical profession has long been accused of paternalism. By this, people mean that doctors come to a conclusion about their patient's condition. They then prescribe a treatment without bothering to involve that patient in the decision. This is now seen to be extremely arrogant. After all, don't we have a right to be informed about all possible options and potential side-effects? And, why should other people tell you what to do, as their views and values may be very different from your own?

This is a central feature of our choice-filled society, where there is a tendency to permit different people to hold their own sets of values and come to their own conclusions. We live in a culture of choice, where we value very highly the freedom of individuals to make their own decisions.

This sounds very nice in theory—until you think about it. In a perfect, post-modern system, members of the medical profession would act as impartial agents simply obeying their patients' wishes. They would play no directive role in making the final decision. For example, if asked to arrange a heart transplant, it would be their duty to supply it.

So, doctors are now supposed to operate a system of informed consent. Under this regime, a doctor assesses the situation and then discusses the various options available with the woman. She is now supposed to understand everything (i.e. she is informed), and is then asked to choose the treatment path that she wants to follow (i.e. she chooses and gives consent).

In practice, this seldom happens. Faced with some of the hardest decisions she has had to make in her life, she often actively seeks directive advice from her doctor and asks what course of action he or she would recommend. Often the doctor replies by saying that, 'If you were a close friend I would suggest... but it has to be your decision.'

In effect, we have privatized decision-making. You end up

running your life by your own set of principles—and I run mine by my set. The state, rather than providing a guiding or controlling influence, has stepped to one side. The rationale is that the woman needs to make the decision, because it is the woman who has to live with the outcome.

Anyway, health professionals are there to advise you, but at the end of the day when it comes to any tests or procedures on an unborn baby the law states that any decisions rest with the woman. The father may be consulted, but he has no authority over the decision. The law's provision for the woman to have the final say is largely to protect her in a situation where she is in conflict with the baby's father. If the couple is communicating well, the reality is that the decisions, and the responsibility for those decisions, will be shared.

It is also worth noting that not only have we privatized decision-making, we have also privatized the provision of care. The increased costs of looking after a child who needs constant attention will place a formidable strain on any family budget. This leaves many couples facing the option of an abortion or severe financial hardship. Civilized societies should be marked by their desire to care for those in their midst who need most help. Any call to think twice about screening for fetal abnormalities should be accompanied by an offer of assistance from the public purse.

Two types of decision

Couples are faced with two types of decision. The first is which tests to have. The second addresses what to do in the light of the information that the tests provide. If you don't want to do anything with the result of a particular test, it is much better if you do not take the test in the first place.

Both sets of decisions are often made in a hurry. Pregnancy doesn't wait while you have a long, hard think and some tests need to be done at specific times during the pregnancy. People are also very aware that abortions performed early are less traumatic for everyone involved than those done when the developing baby is older. On top of this, UK law is much less stringent about abortions before 24 weeks of pregnancy than any that take place afterwards. But the pressure is on, as many of the results won't be known until after the 20th week. The result is that women can be under distinct pressure to make a quick decision about what course of action to pursue after receiving their test results.

Of course, the ideal scenario is to have considered all of this before getting pregnant. But this rarely occurs, and in any case your views may easily change once you realize the amazing fact that there is a baby on board!

As we have said, any advice given by health professionals is supposed to be strictly non-directive. You should be given information and not instructions. The 1996 survey carried out by the National Childbirth Trust shows that for some people the reality is very different. Ten per cent of the women interviewed felt pressurized in some way. Others reported that their decisions were simply not accepted, or that screening was presented as a routine matter and it was difficult to refuse. Still others reported that their blood samples had been sent for screening tests although they had requested that this should not happen. Some found that they had been booked in for amniocentesis tests before they even knew the results of the screening test. Still others felt pressurized into having an amniocentesis.

Status

Before you can make decisions about which tests you will have, and what you will do with the results, you need to consider what you think is the status of the baby. Until recently, babies have grown inside their mothers' wombs in worlds that were closed to view from the outside world. The result was a level of discussion characterized more by ignorance than information. At times, you have to wonder if anything has changed, as you can still hear people involved in public debates describe the developing baby as a ball of cells, or a lump of jelly.

Lennart Nilsson's photographs, published in 1965, arguably marked the moment that the light was turned on. In his now classic book, *A Child is Born*, photo after photo showed the intricate detail of extremely young embryos and fetuses. From early in development, what we see is a little human being. This wasn't lost on ancient scholars, who called the developing human a 'fetus', the Latin word meaning 'offspring', from just nine weeks after fertilization. After all, by this point all the organs are formed.

The ultrasound scanner has now personalized this information by allowing couples to see an image of their own baby. One doctor, who sees ultrasound scans of babies most weeks of his working life, was surprised by the emotion and elation he felt on seeing his own baby for the first time—this baby was real, this baby was his offspring.

So, with the baby in sight, we are forced to make educated decisions. While science has given us screening, it has also sharpened the focus of the debate.

The decisions that you make will be strongly influenced by your beliefs about the moral value of the unborn baby, and whether you see the unborn child as a current or future member of your family. Taking the last point first, it is all too easy to see birth as the initiation ceremony when an animate object becomes a human being. This view says that prior to birth we have a fetus, an unborn baby; after birth we have a child, an heir. This view arises out of historical ignorance of the life of the unborn child—birth seemed like the start. I don't wish to demean the wonder of birth, but isn't this endowing the event with too much status? Developmentally, little has changed from the baby's point of view and if the baby is a member of your family when he or she is born, then surely he or she was equally a member of your family before the birth?

In Chapter 2 we reviewed the various stages in physical development that may help us to make a judgment about when a human being begins. However, as I indicated then, they all fall short of a definite proof that life starts at that particular point. The basic problem is that each looks for the arrival of a particular function (for example, the start of nerve activity, or higher brain function) and then says, 'Now the embryo is human.' However, this limits the understanding of what it is to be a person to single attributes of capability. The flaw in this approach can be seen, as it leads to ruling out people with particular disabilities who may never achieve these functions.

The one thing that most philosophers and theologians agree on is that we must all tread carefully before claiming to hold the position of absolute truth. However, people have to go on living and so have to adopt positions from which they can operate. In this case, you have to decide when you think a human life starts. As far as I can see, the options all fall into one of three categories.

Category 1: Full human status begins at conception

This is the position taken by many religious groups, including the Roman Catholic Church and some groups within the Protestant evangelical traditions. Their basic argument is that conception is the unique starting-point for every individual's life. From that point on, we have a developing human being. The fact that that person is not capable of performing many activities is of no importance. He or she has intrinsic value because he or she is made and valued by God. The key factor is God's relationship with this new individual, and that is not dependent on the individual's performance of any particular function.

Some people who have no particular religious conviction also join in and point to the potential present in a developing embryo. The argument is that an embryo demands the full status of a human being because it has the potential to live after birth. A newborn baby is basically as helpless as an embryo—left alone, both will die—so if you are going to give full status to a newborn, then why not give it to an embryo?

They also point to the fact that fertilization is the only unique process that could mark a change in a person's status. There is no other stage when you can say, 'Yesterday, it was a piece of biological material, but today he is human'. From conception to death there is a continuous process of development and change, with abilities being gained and lost along the way.

The consequence of holding this viewpoint is that you can only perform actions on an embryo or fetus that are ethically allowable on an individual after birth. That rules out abortion in all but the most extreme circumstances, where to leave the embryo seriously endangers the mother's life. The option then is to stand by and watch both die, or to act and at least save the mother.

Category 2: Full human status is gradually acquired during pregnancy

It strikes me that most people try to fit somewhere into this group. That doesn't necessarily mean that they are right; could it be that this is simply the most comfortable position to adopt?

The basic thinking is that it seems irrational to say that an embryo consisting of 1, 2, 4, 8, 16, 32, 64... or any easily countable number of cells can have the same status as a fully functioning baby. This then extends to say that the more developed the person becomes, the greater his or her status. It also leads into the argument that an embryo that is clearly going to give rise to a baby who has some severe abnormality is of less value than one that will develop into an apparently fully healthy baby. Similar arguments are sometimes applied to adults with disabilities.

The acquisition of personhood becomes tied to two features. First, there is the baby's ability to perform more and more functions. The questions then are: which functions are of such fundamental importance, and when does the baby acquire them? Secondly, as the baby grows the relationship between parents and child also grows.

This position leaves open the option of performing some actions on a fetus that might be unacceptable on a baby or an adult. The problem is that you are left having to decide just how much or how little value you want to attribute to any particular stage. With no fixed markers, it is very tempting to let these values ebb and flow to suit the individual situation you are faced with.

Category 3: Full human status is achieved at live birth

The legal position in the UK is that each individual acquires the full status of a human being with his or her first breath. A baby who is born after 28 weeks of the pregnancy and dies without taking a breath is recorded as being stillborn but the birth must be notified and a birth certificate is issued. A baby who takes even one breath is the legal heir of any estate, even if he or she dies.

As we mentioned in Chapter 2 this position is getting harder to defend now that special care baby units successfully look after babies who are as young as 24 weeks old. Such infants acquire the full status of a human being and protection of the law some 16 weeks before babies born at the more usual 40 weeks. As far as I can see, this legal structure survives basically because it is administratively convenient.

Status of people with an abnormality

Behind the whole notion of screening for fetal abnormality is the idea that we want to choose not to have a child with a disability. One of the first questions to ask if a test shows an abnormality is whether this is going to lead to any pronounced disability. Many do not.

By having these tests we are faced with having to decide which diseases or abnormalities are so bad that you can justify terminating that life. Would you classify a severely disfiguring harelip or cleft palate in that group? Some do. Would you limit it to conditions that are fatal at birth or in early childhood? This is more common. How about extending it to include diseases that are fatal in mid-life? This is seldom possible at the moment, but it will not be long before genetic screening can identify those with a greater chance of dying early.

Some argue vehemently that even looking for abnormalities is a slur on people who have disabilities. Others say that the tests don't dismiss disabled people who are already in existence; they just give the choice to avoid having any more.

Your reactions

Where you decide that life starts is going to influence your decisions. If you are a member of category 1, then your choices will be limited. You may ask for no tests at all and thus avoid having to make any supplementary decisions.

You may ask to have any tests that are not designed solely to identify conditions for which there is no treatment. For example the AFP screening test looks for Down's syndrome and spina bifida and nothing else. If you have no intention of aborting your baby then you may well choose to avoid these. But the ultrasound scan can reveal the position of the placenta or other treatable physical conditions, as well as other physical abnormalities (see chapter 6). Such information may increase the doctors' ability to provide care for your unborn baby.

Finally, you may decide to have all of the tests. If an abnormality is detected you will then have time to prepare yourself and your family for the task of bringing up a child with a special need.

You may still wish to avoid an amniocentesis or CVS which bring with them a high risk of a miscarriage. If you agree with the arguments in categories 2 and 3 then you will be faced with a wider range of options. You can still avoid all testing, but are more likely to start with any tests that do not directly endanger the baby's life. Then come the results...

Faced with the results of your screening tests, you have to answer two questions: first, in your own mind does the result indicate so high a risk that your baby has some abnormality that you want to take some action? Remember that the screening tests will almost never give definite answers; you will be presented the information in the form of a probability, a chance. If your answer is no then you need progress no further. However do remember that this hasn't guaranteed you a healthy baby—it has simply eliminated a few possibilities.

'I had let them do the blood test without really thinking about the consequences and without realizing that I could have refused it.'

If you believe that there is a substantial risk of an abnormality, you are faced with the second decision, as you choose between the four basic courses. Are you going to have more tests, terminate the pregnancy, prepare yourself for life with a disabled child, or try to treat the condition while the baby is in the womb?

More tests

As the screening blood tests only give results in the form of a probability, you will be offered a CVS or amniocentesis which give a more definite result. There are two key drawbacks to both

e tests. First, each carries a significant risk of causing a
rriage. This means that in trying to see whether your baby
ealthy the procedure may bring the pregnancy to an abrupt
end. The question you need to ask yourself is, are you prepared
to take that risk? If your purpose in having the tests is to
determine whether you wish to continue with the pregnancy
then you may feel that the risks are acceptable. If you decide that
the risk of the test is too high, you will then have to live out the
rest of your pregnancy with a nagging anxiety over your baby's
health. In this case you may well find yourself regretting having
the initial test.

Secondly, even if the test comes back showing some genetic or
chromosomal disorder it will rarely tell you how severely the
baby is affected by the condition. You are still left making critical
decisions with very limited information.

Abort

The main reason why the issue of antenatal screening is so
emotive and controversial is that the tests seldom detect diseases
that can be cured. This makes them very unusual, as it is
considered unethical to offer screening tests when no treatment
is available. The implication is that an abortion is the treatment.

This is not the place to describe the range of abortion
techniques commonly used. Suffice it to say that all are
unpleasant for everyone involved. The older the unborn child,
the more unpleasant the process.

Out of 154,315 terminations of pregnancy in England and
Wales in 1995, 301 were because the developing baby had
Down's syndrome, 166 had anencephaly, 144 had spina bifida
and 68 had hydrocephalus. A further 1,144 abortions were
performed because the unborn baby had one or more of a wide
range of physical abnormalities.

Looking at newspapers and watching recent TV programmes,

I believe that there is a growing sense of unease in society at the moment about the number of abortions carried out each year. Most of this stems from the perception that all too often abortion is used almost as a form of contraception. However, it is unfair to group all abortions together. People who choose to abort an unhealthy baby normally do so with great uncertainty and anguish.

Because tests take time and some can only be conducted relatively late in a pregnancy, babies can be quite well formed at the time of the abortion. In the UK, abortions are allowed up until term if a severe abnormality is detected. This is a controversial piece of legislation, partly because there is no definition of what constitutes a severe handicap.

As the recent survey conducted by the National Childbirth Trust indicated (see page 51), all too often members of the medical profession assume that a couple will ask for an abortion if a handicap is detected. The suggestion is made that a couple is being irresponsible in bringing a disabled child into the world. He or she will place an unacceptable burden on society. 'After all,' they say, 'you may decide to devote yourselves to looking after this child, but what will happen when you are old or die?' The implication is that no one else will be prepared to assist in providing care. This is a sad reflection on our society, but at the moment it is a real problem.

Prepare

A strong argument in favour of screening tests is that they give the couple time to prepare themselves, their family and their home. They also allow the medical profession to ensure that specialists are on hand at the baby's birth so that the best available care can be given.

However, this argument has a weakness if the tests are not capable of giving definite answers. There are numerous examples

> '*It seemed that each individual decision we took made sense by itself, but when you look at the whole experience it was a series of escalating interventions—just what we had wanted to avoid.*'

of couples who have had an agonizing six or so months after a screening test indicated that their baby was at an increased risk of some abnormality, only to find, when the baby is born, that all is OK. Let's face it, if you take a group of 10 people who have been given a 1 in 10 chance of their baby having some problem, then on average nine of them are going to find that the anxiety was all in vain.

If the tests indicate some definite problem, such as a missing limb or heart malformation, then couples can spend the rest of their pregnancy adjusting their expectations. In some ways, this turns the pregnancy into a time of grieving, grieving the loss of your original dream of a healthy family. However, it does mean that by the time the baby is born you will have started to come to terms with the situation. As part of this process you will have had the opportunity to contact other families with similarly affected children and to get in touch with any self-help and support groups in your area.

Treat

The other benefit that can come from screening programmes is the ability to treat some conditions. Currently, surgery before birth is rare, but if you argue that a person's life starts at conception, then that person should be offered the best medical support from that day onwards. (The treatments of specific conditions are discussed in chapter 7.)

Beware the screening roller-coaster

Simply going with the flow and accepting the first screening tests is the easy option—it's only another blood test. But many couples have found that they are soon unwittingly drawn into a sequence of tests that they had no intention of having, but don't feel able to turn down.

There is no quick fix. The only option is to consider the whole implication of screening tests before having the first one. No health professional should expect, or even allow, you to take a screening test without ensuring that you understand exactly what you are doing. Your comprehension of the test and the nature of the results that it will generate lies at the heart of informed consent. The golden rule is that if you are uncertain about anything, then ask—and keep asking until you get a satisfactory answer.

Long-term implications

Whatever decision you take has implications that you will have to live with for the rest of your life. Some are more momentous than others.

A decision not to have tests

If you are considering turning down the offer of tests then you also need to consider the implications. You must realize that in doing this you have decided to rule out the possibility of dealing with some conditions that can be managed better if they are discovered, or even treated, before birth. You may feel that screening tests which only give a probability of disability, such as the Bart's or Leeds tests, can be turned down, because they indicate conditions for which the sole treatment is an abortion. In so doing, you also turn down the ability to have time to come to terms with the situation. An ultrasound scan, on the other hand, can occasionally identify conditions where knowing about the abnormality before birth can be a great advantage.

A few conditions, such as blocked tubes running to and from the bladder, can be treated surgically before birth, and others, such as heart defects and umbilical hernias, can often be sorted out very successfully immediately after birth. In all of these situations, advance warning is beneficial to the baby. Apart from anything else, it gives time for the mother to go to a specialist centre for the delivery so that the baby can be given the best expert care. This is much better than rushing the baby off in an ambulance for treatment at a major hospital as soon as he or she is born, leaving the mother recovering from the delivery in a local hospital many miles away.

Advance warning that the placenta is blocking the baby's exit from the womb—'placenta praevia'—can save lives. The placenta is low in the womb, or blocks the birth canal, in about 1 in 200 pregnancies. The condition can cause massive bleeding in late pregnancy. It also indicates that the baby will need to be born by Caesarean section a couple of weeks early, to avoid the mother going into natural labour which would be extremely dangerous.

On a less dramatic scale, an ultrasound can also confirm the date of the pregnancy to within a week and detect whether the baby is growing at an appropriate speed. If the baby stops growing, then doctors may recommend that it would be best for the baby to be born and cared for in a special-care baby unit. While this is not ideal, it may be better than leaving the baby in the womb.

If you decide to turn down this opportunity, you need to

realize that you will deny your baby the possibility of beneficial treatments. There is the chance that you may have to live with the thought that if you had had the scan, things might have worked out differently.

Living with a child who has an abnormality

Not all abnormalities have a severe effect on the person's life. An abnormality where the baby is found to have an extra X chromosome (i.e. 47, XXX; see chapter 7) will only result in very mild learning difficulties. This highlights the importance of talking with a trained counsellor who can help you understand the implications of any particular abnormality.

A child with a severe disability will change your family, particularly if you already have a child. But don't forget, your family changes irrevocably whenever another child is born. However, a disabled child will undoubtedly need and demand hours of attention each day. You will have to make room in your life for this. Your careers, holidays, hobbies and time available for other members of your family will all be affected. Most couples who have such babies find that life doesn't stop, but it does take a new direction.

One of the hardest things is that while able-bodied children

'At first I regretted taking the test because I was going to proceed regardless of the results. Later, I realized that advance knowledge of any problems could help my baby.'

normally leave home and lead their own lives at the end of their teens, a disabled child may need care and attention for many more years. For the parents of these children, the natural post-kids life, where you can regain freedom and spontaneity, may never occur.

The provision for disabled people in our society is inadequate. So it will often be up to the parents to push for physiotherapy, special schooling and any other special needs. Many of these facilities will have to be paid for by the parents.

Post-abortion trauma

Many couples find that the trauma of an abortion does not end when the woman has recovered from the physical procedure. Many need long-term support and counselling over months, maybe even years. You may need to talk about the tragedy, or may become withdrawn and feel isolated. Support agencies like SATFA and CARE find that from time to time people experience feelings of guilt, failure, jealousy, anger or blame towards other family members.

People who have an abortion because the baby has some handicap tend to be particularly severely affected and take longer to recover emotionally from the experience than those who abort an unplanned and unwanted pregnancy. This, after all, is a much-wanted baby, who the couple hoped would become a member of their family. Couples are suffering not only the trauma of the procedure but also grieving the loss of a child.

Talking with your partner is often very hard, though it is essential that throughout this time you maintain a strong relationship. Ask for help from professionals if you feel unable to cope—this is a sign of concern for your relationship, not a sign of weakness. Some GP surgeries and churches can direct you to specially trained counsellors who can assist you and help you understand your own feelings.

Some health professionals claim that there are benefits for couples with a child that is expected to die at birth, who decide not to have an abortion and to continue pregnancy to term, even though this may involve another three months of pregnancy. They then experience the birth and hold their baby. These couples meet their baby and are then in a better position to grieve the loss. Most are surprised that the physical abnormalities are not as frightening to see as they had imagined and find the experience comforting. Parents often spot familial resemblances and make comments such as, 'Look, he's got Uncle Joe's nose.' Photographs taken at this point can also be a focus for grieving and even a source of comfort. A midwife will be very willing to take some, so that you have a record of this member of your family. No one is pretending that seeing or holding your baby is going to be easy, but where it is possible it can be helpful.

Summary

The most important thing is that you know why you are having any particular test *before* you take it. If you realize that you won't want to do anything with the results of an individual test, let your health team know that you don't want the test. They may check that you understand what you are doing, but they should not try to override your decision.

Mike and Sue

Mike and Sue are both practising Christians. They found it very hard to convince their consultant that they didn't want any screening tests, even though Sue was 45 years old.

For three years, Sue and her husband Mike had explored the possibility of using fertility treatments to get their dreamt-for child. As Sue was over 40, they were told that there was little hope of her eggs ever leading to a healthy child and, having thought about it, they were not willing to contemplate egg donation. Then, at the age of 45, Sue suddenly found to her joy that she was pregnant. Her consultant was extremely concerned, as she was the oldest first-time mother he had dealt with.

Mike is a lecturer at a Bible college and the couple's Christian faith strongly influenced the decisions they took throughout the pregnancy.

'When we told my consultant the good news that I was pregnant, he was shocked and horrified,' says Sue. 'The first thing he wrote in my notes was "1 in 32 chance of abnormality". There was a tangible feeling of panic as he asked me to lie on the couch, so that he could have a look at the baby using ultrasound, convinced that at my age he was going to find an abnormal baby. We were 13 weeks into the pregnancy and the baby on the screen looked fine. Everyone relaxed—a little.

'He then talked to us about whether we wanted to go through further tests. Because if there was anything wrong, the earlier the termination the better. We turned down the tests, but he was insistent that we came back for a scan at 18–20 weeks. I didn't realize at that stage that the mid-term scan was to look specifically for abnormalities. I just thought it was to check on development and that sort of thing. During the scan, it dawned on me exactly what was going on and in retrospect I am annoyed that I was put through it basically against my will.

'I knew very strongly that only God can give life. So if God gave life and it was not according to what we would call healthy, then that was the life he had given. I think we were convinced that this was the life that we have been given to nurture and that we would love and look after him or her, come what may. I don't think that I could have had a termination, even if the scan had shown that my baby had no brain; I certainly didn't see Down's syndrome as something worthy of a termination. We also knew that some of the tests were risky—and any risk was too great. Mike had lived next door to a family with a child who had a severe learning difficulty and his parents looked after him well into his 30s or 40s. Mike had thus learned from personal experience that people with disabilities can still lead fulfilled lives.

'For the next six months I became the consultant's prize guinea pig—his oldest first-time mother. Everybody in the clinic knew me and at every visit he had found more reasons to be concerned, more tests to recommend. As I was seeing him every fortnight from 20 weeks, and then at weekly intervals from 30 weeks, this was a lot of concern to handle, a lot of tests to turn down.

'At 20 weeks I started bleeding and was rushed to hospital. Everyone in sight was telling me that I was probably going to lose the baby. They couldn't get the ultrasound scan machine to work, they couldn't work the heart-rate monitor. In the midst of all the tension I burst out laughing—I was convinced that God was in control and was far more powerful than the medics and all their machinery. Their hope was in their machine, my hope was in God.

'At 30 weeks my blood pressure went up a little, spawning another session of doom and gloom. Then they thought that the child was growing too fast and they panicked again that I might have gestational diabetes and I was sent to see a dietitian. I had an excellent diet. Even so, I was booked in to see the nutritionist. I went without complaint, not realizing that I was going to be put through an hour-long interrogation. By the end of it I thought that if I munched a digestive biscuit I would kill my baby! I started gearing myself up to the idea that this child was not going to be healthy.

'At 34 weeks they started talking about how long the pregnancy should go on—I was becoming a crumbling wreck. The consultant was visibly unhappy after 36 weeks and suggested a Caesarean. At 38 weeks they were worried. The registrar said that they didn't feel that they had the nerve to sit this out. It was them, not us, who were panicking.

'At 40 weeks they did induce me. It was a horrible delivery, but I gave birth to a wonderful, healthy daughter.

'In fairness to the medical team, this was a very much desired baby and they were doing everything, everything to make sure that we had a good outcome. I respect them for that, but I didn't feel that I was being allowed to make my decisions. I was simply in the hands of medical science.

'The idea that we were prepared to turn down testing was utterly incredible to the medical staff; they just couldn't come to terms with it. Two days after the birth the midwife sat on the end of my bed and said, "Next time you will have tests, won't you? This time you were lucky, but don't risk it next time." Even then, they still wouldn't accept our decision not to have tests.'

Notes

1. A. Clarke and E.P. Parsons, Institute of Medical Genetics, University of Wales College of Medicine.

5

Checking on the mother's health

Some tests examine the woman's health and check that nothing goes wrong during her pregnancy. These are routine and normally demand no particular response. They give no information about the growing baby.

An expanding range of tests is now offered during pregnancy. It is part of an extensive range of screening programmes that are used to uncover people who are in the early stages of a disease. Some tests check that the woman is keeping well and that nothing starts to go wrong during her pregnancy. These are routine and normally demand no particular response. Other tests are directed at the developing baby, aiming to see whether the baby is fundamentally healthy.

Your initial tests are made during the initial 'booking visit', which often happens at home when a community midwife visits you. The midwife will probably record your weight and measure your height. Together, these help the healthcare team to assess whether you are likely to have a small pelvis and therefore may need extra assistance at the delivery. They also give a baseline measurement from which your midwife may spot any large weight changes during your pregnancy, which could indicate some problem.

The midwife will collect blood in a series of tubes. Somewhat gruesomely they are called the 'booking bloods' and will be sent to a laboratory for a routine series of tests:

Early tests

Blood group

The tests will check your blood group, to see which of the major blood groups you belong to—A, B, AB or O. This will be recorded in your notes so that an appropriate pack of blood can be found without any delay if at any point in the pregnancy or birth you need a transfusion.

Rhesus factor

As well as belonging to one of the major blood groups, everyone's blood is either Rhesus positive or Rhesus negative. Blood cells are coated with many different proteins called antigens. One, called 'factor D', is present in the blood of seven out of eight people. These people are said to have Rhesus positive blood. The remaining one in eight Rhesus negative people have no factor D.

Problems start when a woman who has Rhesus negative blood gives birth to a baby whose blood is Rhesus positive (Figure 2(a)), which can only occur if her partner is Rhesus positive. In the UK this occurs in about one in 11 pregnancies. If both partners are Rhesus negative there should be no problem. During labour, as the placenta starts to break away from the womb, small amounts of the baby's blood enter the mother's circulation (Figure 2 (b)). The factor D in the baby's blood is recognized as 'foreign' and the mother builds proteins, antibodies, that destroy the baby's

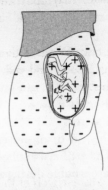

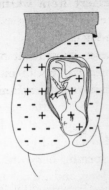

(a) A Rhesus negative mother carries a Rhesus positive baby.

(b) Around birth, some of the baby's blood passes into the mother's circulation.

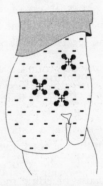

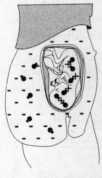

(c) Over the next few days, the mother develops antibodies that attack and destroy the baby's blood cells.

(d) In a subsequent Rhesus positive pregnancy, these antibodies can damage the baby (Rhesus disease).

Figure 2: Rhesus explained

blood (Figure 2(c)). The first baby is seldom harmed, because by the time these antibodies have been made the baby has been born and is safe.

However, subsequent babies are at risk. Without treatment, the antibodies remain in the woman's blood and may attack future unborn babies (Figure 2(d)). This problem can usually be prevented. Soon after giving birth, a Rhesus negative woman is injected with artificial antibodies which destroy any of the baby's blood that entered her circulation. This, in turn, prevents the mother forming her own antibodies. The artificial antibodies do not last long, and are not around to cause trouble during a future pregnancy.

A blood sample taken at the initial booking with the midwife will be analysed to see if it contains red cell antibodies. Rhesus negative women will have another sample taken at 28 weeks and all women have a sample taken at 36 weeks. If any of these are positive for antibodies, then they will be asked to come into the clinic for frequent tests to check if the levels of antibodies are rising or falling.

In the rare cases where the antibody count rises to dangerous levels, doctors may recommend that they collect a sample of the baby's blood to see if anaemia is developing. This is done using a long needle that is passed through the mother's abdomen and womb, and into a vessel in the baby's umbilical cord. Even using ultrasound scanners to guide the needle, the procedure is difficult and not without dangers, because bleeding may occur once the needle has been withdrawn. Just as in amniocentesis and CVS there is also a 1 in 200 risk of a miscarriage after this blood test. If the unborn baby is anaemic, your doctors may recommend that they give the baby a blood transfusion while it is still in the womb. This is described in chapter 8.

A national policy of treating Rhesus negative mothers has reduced the number of cases of Rhesus disease dramatically, but it has not been eradicated. Testing your blood early in pregnancy means that you can be given all of the appropriate treatment at the appropriate times.

Blood count

A blood count determines the number of red blood cells in your blood. These are packed with an iron-containing molecule called haemoglobin that carries oxygen around your body. If you do not have ample iron in your diet, you may develop anaemia and will not be able to carry enough oxygen. A low blood count indicates that you have anaemia.

Anaemia is always a bad thing, but particularly so during pregnancy, when a woman's blood must transport oxygen not only for herself, but also for her baby. If you get anaemic, you may become extremely tired and your baby may not grow properly. Eating plenty of meat, hard-boiled eggs, or green vegetables will help by increasing the amount of iron in your diet. If you are becoming anaemic you may also be given iron tablets to supplement your diet.

Sickle test

Sickle-cell anaemia is an inherited blood disorder that is most common in people with an Afro-Caribbean background. If you are affected, your red blood cells are shaped like a sickle blade rather than a Frisbee, and do not transport oxygen very effectively. You will have a permanent form of anaemia. If appropriate, your blood will be tested to see whether you carry the sickle-cell gene. If so, your partner's blood should also be tested. If both of you carry the gene then your unborn baby has a 1 in 4 chance of being affected and you will be referred to a specialist.

There is no cure for sickle-cell anaemia and, until 30 years ago, almost all children with it died in childhood. With increased levels of basic care, many people with the disorder do survive to adulthood—with varying degrees of symptoms—and some sufferers are having children of their own.

Rubella (German measles)

Your blood will also be analysed to check that you have been successfully immunized against rubella. If so, you and your baby are safe from the disease. If the test shows that you are not protected from this disease, you will be given advice on how to minimize your risk. For one thing, wherever possible you should try to avoid contact with anyone who currently has rubella. Doctors will recommend that you are immunized after you have given birth, to protect you and any babies you may have in the future.

Hepatitis B

A test will also look to see whether you have ever been infected by the hepatitis B virus. If you have, you will be offered an injection for your baby following delivery. The condition is common in some Asian racial groups, but rarely occurs in people from other backgrounds.

Other hepatitis screening may be offered for hepatitis A and C. You should ask for information on these tests if you think you may be at risk—perhaps as a result of foreign travel, or a history of drug abuse.

Syphilis

Another routine test is for syphilis. While this is seldom positive, the disease is easy to treat during pregnancy but, to prevent the disease passing to the baby, any treatment needs to start before the 20th week of pregnancy.

HIV

You can ask for a test for HIV (human immunodeficiency virus), the virus which causes AIDS (acquired immune deficiency syndrome). This should only be given after you have been counselled about the consequences of having the test, and is only needed if you have some reason to suspect that you may be infected with the virus.

Some antenatal clinics perform HIV checks on every woman. Their aim is to see the extent of HIV in the community. Care is taken to ensure that these tests are anonymous so that any individuals cannot be identified.

Ongoing tests

In addition to the one-off tests conducted at the beginning of pregnancy, there is a series of tests that you will be given every time you see your doctor or midwife.

Blood pressure

At each visit to your doctor or midwife, your blood pressure will be monitored. It can change enormously during pregnancy and can give warning of the onset of pre-eclampsia, a condition that is dangerous for both mother and baby (see Glossary).

Urine

Regular checks of the sugar and protein content of the woman's urine should be made throughout pregnancy. If the level of sugar rises, these may be backed up with blood tests.

Sugar in the urine is an indication that the woman may have pregnancy-induced diabetes. Where this occurs it normally starts about halfway through a pregnancy. For some reason, the woman is not producing enough of the hormone insulin to keep her blood sugar levels under control. Insulin is normally released into the bloodstream from the pancreas as the level of glucose rises in a person's blood. This increased insulin makes the body remove glucose from the blood and either use it or store it away. If there is insufficient insulin, glucose concentrations rise and the unborn baby may receive too large a supply of energy, causing excessive growth. This can lead to problems for the baby and mother, not least of which is a difficult birth, as a result of the baby being grossly overweight. In addition to sending too much glucose to the developing baby, some glucose escapes into urine.

Often, gestational diabetes can be controlled by eating carefully. An appointment should be made to see a nutritionist or dietitian, who will be able to give appropriate dietary advice. In more extreme cases the woman may need to start taking insulin. The good news is that as soon as the baby is born the diabetes simply goes away.

Protein in the urine may be a sign of high blood pressure or a kidney infection, both of which would need monitoring carefully.

Abdominal checks

At each visit, your doctor or midwife will feel your tummy to find the top of the womb. This gives a good indication of how well the baby is growing and which way it is lying. As pregnancy progresses you may be able to feel various parts of the baby, such as the head, arms, legs, feet and bottom.

Ankle oedema

The midwife will check for any swelling around your ankle. This is an indication of fluid retention, which can be caused by high blood pressure. If your ankles start to swell you will be given advice to take plenty of rest.

6

Testing the baby's health

There is a growing range of screening and diagnostic tests which try to assess the health of the unborn baby. The tests are based on ultrasound scans, maternal blood samples and samples of the baby's cells.

In addition to routinely listening to the baby's heartbeat at antenatal visits, various tests are now offered to pregnant women to see if the unborn baby is healthy. The first tests are based on the principle of screening and aim to show whether the potential for a problem is greater or less than for an average member of the population. If these tests indicate that you are in a high-risk category for a particular condition then you may be offered a second series of tests. These aim to be more firmly diagnostic. Some tests count the number of chromosomes in the baby's cells. Fully healthy individuals have 46 chromosomes and anything else will lead to some form of disability. At the same time these tests can show whether the unborn baby is a boy or a girl. Other tests look for specific damage to the genes on individual chromosomes.

The exact nature of the tests you are offered varies from hospital to hospital. Make sure you read any leaflets that you are given and always ask if you don't understand something. It is most unlikely that you will ask a question that the doctors, nurses and midwives have not had to answer before.

Ultrasound

From the first dim images of a moving heart that came out of a Rotterdam research base in the late 1960s, ultrasound has rapidly flourished into an everyday medical tool. While it is now used in many areas of medicine, the most well-known clinical application of ultrasound is in obstetrics. Here, it offers expectant parents the first glimpse of their unborn child. The pictures may be a little unclear, particularly to the untrained eye, but it is basically a safe, non-invasive way of observing unborn babies. The image on the screen is a cross section through the mother's abdomen and through the baby. This means that you can see the baby's bones, heart, kidney, brain and almost any other organ.

Within the next decade the clarity of images produced is likely to increase dramatically and there are already some machines that produce three-dimensional ultrasound images. It is fascinating to see a three-dimensional picture of a face that has never seen the light of day.

Ultrasound scans give a picture of the baby. This allows you to observe basic physical features. As the baby develops, an increasing number of physical characteristics can be examined. While this has huge potential, it also has its limitations. The pictures are unclear, the baby may happen to be lying in a position that means that some of it can't be seen, and just because a particular organ is present doesn't mean it is necessarily working properly.

Every now and then a scare blows up in the press that ultrasound scanning can damage the unborn baby. Since we have been told that the scans are safe, such reports understandably cause a stir. The stories have often been based on a few studies that appear to have shown that the more scans an unborn baby is exposed to, the more likely he or she is to have some physical handicap. However, the very people who are most at risk of carrying a child with an abnormality are the people given the largest numbers of scans. It is therefore quite possible that the presence of a problem leads to the number of scans rather than the number of scans leading to the handicap.

Remember that the vast majority of routine ultrasound scans are conducted with the purpose of looking to see if anything is wrong—it's normally called an 'Ultrasound scan for fetal abnormality'. While this is undoubtedly a wonderful opportunity for you to catch a glimpse of your hidden offspring and take home a dim and shady picture to show friends and family, that isn't why the health professionals spend millions of pounds providing this service. The task is to see if there is any indication that your baby may not be developing normally. If you don't want to know whether your baby has a physical abnormality before he or she is born, then think twice before having the scan. Although most health professionals will automatically assume that you want a scan, there is nothing to say that you have to accept the offer. However, read on before you make that decision. A scan can also detect conditions that are dangerous to you or your unborn baby. If you decide to go ahead with the scan, then take time to think about the full purpose of this visit beforehand.

An early scan—often called a dating scan

PREGNANCY STAGE
This scan can be before the sixth week.

PURPOSE
Occasionally, women are offered a scan early in their pregnancy. The most common reason for this is to confirm a pregnancy in patients undergoing fertility treatment. The doctor will want to check that the baby is embedded in the wall of the womb rather than in one of the tubes leading from the ovary to the womb or

on the outside of the womb. At other times, it may be used to date accurately the start of a pregnancy.

The doctor may try to get a better picture by using a small probe passed into the woman's vagina.

There is no strong evidence that ultrasound scanning by itself carries any appreciable risk to the health of the fetus.

WHAT CAN BE SEEN
At this stage the embryo should be just visible, with a flickering pulsation of its heart beating at about 160 beats per minute. As the embryo's length doubles every 10 days from six to nine weeks, a measurement of total length can determine when the egg was fertilized to within six days.

An early scan also allows the healthcare team to count the number of embryos that are developing. This can be particularly important if the woman is involved in some forms of fertility treatment, as high multiple pregnancies lead to a variety of problems. As it is generally accepted that conceiving more than twins is less than ideal, from a medical and psychological point of view (there is a very high risk of triplets being born extremely prematurely and therefore having some handicap. Also, there is no special financial assistance for parents with triplets and no rest for the first few years of the triplets' lives), you may find yourself in the position of being offered a selective abortion. The idea here is to remove one or more embryos and leave you with twins. It is important to bear in mind that selectively aborting some embryos increases the risk of a miscarriage and the subsequent loss of all of the babies.

Scans may also be offered around this stage to investigate the cause of bleeding and confirm whether or not a woman is still pregnant.

King's Down's syndrome screening test

Also called the Nuchal Thickening Test and Nuchal Translucency Test.

PREGNANCY STAGE
Usually performed around 10 to 14 weeks.

PURPOSE
The sole purpose of this test is to look for physical markers that may indicate Down's syndrome or some other chromosomal abnormality.

RISKS
There is no strong evidence that ultrasound scanning by itself carries any appreciable risk to the health of the fetus.

WHAT CAN BE SEEN
You cannot see Down's syndrome on an ultrasound scan, but you can see some physical characteristics that may indicate that the baby has an unusual set of chromosomes.

One of the more recent screening tests to be offered is an ultrasound scan that specifically measures the thickness of skin folds (nuchal folds) around the base of the baby's neck. This can be seen on the scan as a dark area and the ultrasonographer will measure its width in millimetres. If the area is large it shows that fluid is accumulating here (nuchal oedema) and indicates that the baby may have Down's syndrome. A computer will calculate the risk of Down's syndrome by taking account of the age and size of the unborn baby. This test was first identified and used by doctors in King's College Hospital, London, hence its name.

If a larger than expected area is found at the back of the neck, the ultrasonographer will try to look for other associated markers, such as an increased gap between the baby's big and second toes, as well as heart defects.

This test does not give a definite yes or no to the question: 'Does my baby have Down's syndrome?' It is only a screening test that gives an indication of the situation. A 'positive' result means that the baby is at increased risk of having Down's syndrome, a 'negative' result means that he or she is not at an increased risk. However, some health authorities are starting to use this means of screening instead of AFP, Bart's or Leeds tests because they believe it gives more definite results. As a result, its use is likely to become more widespread.

Mid-pregnancy screening scan

PREGNANCY STAGE
Somewhere between 18 to 22 weeks is now commonly accepted as the time for the first 'routine' scan.

PURPOSE
The full title for this scan reveals its main purpose; it is an ultrasound scan for fetal abnormality. The idea is to look to see that the unborn baby is physically healthy before the pregnancy goes past the 24 week date. In addition it is a good opportunity to look for a multiple pregnancy of twins, triplets or more and check the position of the placenta.

RISKS
There is no strong evidence that ultrasound scanning by itself carries any appreciable risk to the health of the fetus.

WHAT CAN BE SEEN
By 20 weeks the unborn baby is large enough for a fairly thorough examination of the baby's anatomy. At this stage, the length of the baby's upper leg bone, the femur, and the diameter of his head can be measured and used to check the date of the pregnancy. The ultrasonographer will only recommend that the

estimated due date is altered if the date that these measurements suggest is more than two weeks greater or less than the original estimate.

Singleton, twins or more
One of the first things an ultrasonographer does is check how many babies are growing inside. It can come as an enormous shock to some couples to be told they have twins, but 1 in 80 pregnancies conceived naturally are twin pregnancies and 1 in 6,400 are triplets. Some fertility treatments substantially increase the chance of a multiple pregnancy, up to a chance of 1 in 4 for twins.

Almost three-quarters of twins are non-identical. This means that they developed from two separate eggs fertilized by two different sperm. The remaining one-quarter of twins are genetically identical, having started out as a single egg that divided early in development. The ultrasound scan may be able to tell you straight away whether or not they are identical, or you may have to wait until they are born.

If you have twins you may well be invited back for extra scans, as it is more difficult for the doctors and midwives to monitor how well the babies are growing just by feeling them. Nearer to the time of delivery it is also more difficult to work out which way each of them is lying, so again a scan can provide useful information.

Healthy placenta
The placenta is a structure that is attached to the wall of the womb. It forms the physical communication between mother and unborn baby, allowing oxygen and nutrients to pass to the baby and many of the baby's waste products to pass back to the mother for her to dispose of.

As the baby grows, the placenta's task increases and so it also needs to grow. In fact the baby and his or her placenta are fairly similar sizes. The main cause for concern is if the placenta positions itself low in the womb. In some cases, the placenta may be so low in the womb that it will prevent the baby getting out. Advance warning of this situation again is worthwhile, as it allows doctors to plan ahead and for the baby to be born by a Caesarean section before the woman goes into labour.

On the other hand the placenta may actually grow right over the birth canal. As the mother's blood flows freely under the placenta this means that if her cervix opens at all during the pregnancy or labour there is the distinct possibility of a severe haemorrhage. These can be extremely serious so any warning of the situation is more than useful. Women in this situation often spend the last few weeks of their pregnancy in bed, often in hospital. The baby will probably need to be delivered by a Caesarean.

Poor fetal growth

Ultrasound scanners are equipped with technology that enables them to make precise measurements of the unborn baby. The two standard measurements are the length of the femur and the diameter of the skull around the forehead. Measurements are then compared with tables that show the range of expected values for a baby of that age.

If the baby is significantly smaller than expected this indicates one of two things. Either the woman's dates are wrong and the baby is younger than expected, or the baby is not growing as well as would be expected. Doctors call this *in utero* growth retardation, or IUGR. You will probably be asked to come back in a week or two for a second scan. If the baby has grown well between the scan then there is nothing to worry about, but you may have to readjust your due date. If the baby has not grown as much as would be expected you will be referred to a consultant for further tests.

Volume of liquid around your baby

The liquid surrounding the baby appears black on the ultrasound scan. Doctors have developed charts that allow them to measure the deepest pool of fluid and estimate the total volume of fluid—they sometimes call it 'liquor'. The volume varies from woman to woman, and from one pregnancy to the next. On average, at 10 weeks of pregnancy there is around 25 ml (1 fl oz), but by 20 weeks this has risen to around 600 ml (about 1 pint). After 36 weeks of pregnancy there will be about 1,200 ml (2 pints) of fluid surrounding the baby. Then over the last few weeks before the baby is born the amount of fluid tends to reduce.

Occasionally, a woman may have too much fluid in the womb—doctors call this polyhydramnios, or conversely there is too little fluid—called oligohydramnios. Both of these can be picked up in a routine scan.

If there is too much fluid, this may point to the baby having some problem that is preventing him or her swallowing the fluid. The fluid is not recycled so it builds up in the womb. The major problem is that it can lead to a premature labour as the womb gets stretched. It also gives the baby too much room for movement later in pregnancy, putting him or her at risk of tangling in the umbilical cord and not settling head down in the birth canal, making for a tricky delivery.

Too little fluid can affect lung development and may indicate a problem with the baby's kidneys or bladder. It could also indicate that the placenta is not performing its job properly.

Kidneys

Kidney problems are not uncommon. They can be picked up on an ultrasound scan and are normally not serious. In fact, most correct themselves without treatment and often before the baby is born.

A few conditions, however, are persistent. Sometimes the tubes running from the kidney to the bladder or from the bladder to the outside are absent or blocked. As a result, pressure builds up in the kidney, which can cause long-term damage or death. A routine ultrasound check will see that the kidneys or bladder are the wrong shape and you should be advised to see a specialist, as there may be ways of treating the problem before the baby is born (see chapter 8). It may be that the problem is best left until after the birth.

In more extreme situations, one or both kidneys may be missing. It is quite possible for a person to lead a perfectly healthy life with one kidney, but if both kidneys are absent the baby will survive for only a few hours after birth. If this is the case you should be offered counselling to help you think through the implications and the decisions you will need to make.

Heart defects
One in every 100 babies is born with some form of heart defect. Most of these are extremely minor. The time when these are most likely to be picked up is at a scan between 16 and 20 weeks. Even then, the minor defects are unlikely to be seen.

On rare occasions the heart may be too big or too small, or have the wrong number of chambers. If the ultrasonographer believes she has seen something that does not quite look right, she may well book an appointment for you to see a consultant obstetrician with special expertise in ultrasound scanning.

If a problem is found, doctors may recommend that you also have an amniocentesis to see if there is any gross genetic abnormality. This may help reveal the exact nature of the problem. If a heart defect is spotted during pregnancy, a paediatric heart specialist should be on hand at the delivery to examine the baby as soon as he or she is born.

The important factor is to identify serious problems where early surgery can be life saving. Arrangements can then be made for you to deliver the baby in a hospital where specialized surgery is available at birth.

Problems that need immediate surgery are rare and most can wait for weeks or months until the baby has grown and is stronger.

Make sure you ask all the questions that you have and continue asking until you understand all that you feel you need to know.

Club foot

About one baby in every 900 is born with a foot twisted out of shape or position. There are many different types of deformity, but together the medical term for this condition is 'talipes'.

The reason why this occurs is unknown. There may be some genetic link, or it may be that there were unusual pressures placed on the foot by the way the baby was lying in the womb.

The most common form of the condition is called talipes equinovarus. The heel is turned inwards and the rest of the foot is bent down. The shin-bone may be twisted and there may be poor development of some of the leg muscles. The problem is twice as common in boys as in girls, and in half of the cases it affects both feet. There is no way of treating the condition before birth, but again antenatal screening may detect it and give you time to get used to the idea that your baby is going to need extra care. With appropriate treatment in the first few years, this should not cause any long-term problems.

Cleft lip and palate

In the UK around 1 in 850 babies is born with a cleft palate, or lip, or both. Of every nine affected babies, two have only a cleft lip, three have only a cleft palate and four have both. Cleft lips are more common in boys and cleft palates more common in girls. It appears that there may be some genetic factor in the condition, as affected children often have a close family member with one or other condition.

A cleft lip is a vertical split in the upper lip. The split is usually off-centre, though occasionally it is in the middle and is then properly called a 'hare lip'. It may be as minor as a little notch in the lip, or can extend from the gum up to the nose.

A cleft palate is a gap running along the middle of the roof of the mouth—the palate. In severe cases it can run the length of the palate, making a long opening between the mouth and nasal passages. Many people with cleft palates also have hearing difficulties and some have other abnormalities.

The exact problems that cause the two conditions are different. However, both occur during the second and third months of pregnancy when blocks of tissue that form the mouth and face fail to move and join together properly.

While either of these conditions can be detected during an ultrasound scan, all babies should be routinely checked immediately after birth. Babies with a cleft lip are normally able to breast-feed, although babies with a cleft palate will need to be fed using a bottle with a special teat. Surgery is usually carried out when the baby is three months old to repair cleft lips and often leaves no major scar. Cleft palates are generally surgically repaired within 12 months.

If you face the shock of discovering that your baby may have a cleft lip or palate, remember that the prospects for the child having a full recovery and a healthy life are excellent.

Spina bifida
One child in every 1,000 born is affected by some degree of spina bifida. The term refers to a range of conditions in which the nerves that make up the spinal cord bulge through the bones that make up the spine or vertebrae. The condition is frequently accompanied by hydrocephalus, in which fluid accumulates in the head, preventing the brain developing properly.

The condition can be extremely mild or very severe and the effect it has depends on the size of the opening in the vertebra(e), the location of the opening, and the amount of damage that has been caused to the spinal cord and brain. A small defect low in the back may cause no problems, or mild leg weakness and poor sensation. Larger defects in the spine can lead to paralysis of the legs and loss of control of the bladder and bowel.

After 16 weeks of pregnancy most cases of spina bifida should be detectable at a routine ultrasound scan. If this is the case the ultrasonographer will find that the tissue that forms the spine has not folded into a complete tube. If the scan shows any uncertainty then you may be recommended to have a blood test to measure the levels of alpha-fetoprotein (see later in this chapter, page 91).

Watching blood flow

Many ultrasound scanners are equipped with technology that allows the ultrasonographer to measure the speed of blood moving in arteries and veins. The way it works is very similar to the police speed guns that bounce a radar signal off a moving car. In the ultrasound scanner, sound waves are bounced off moving blood cells.

This technique is rarely carried out as part of a routine scan, but it can be used to give valuable information about the health of the placenta. It can also help doctors make decisions about the best way to proceed in a situation where the baby is not growing as rapidly as they would otherwise have expected.

A similar examination can be carried out on the artery that supplies maternal blood to the womb, the uterine artery, and thereby supplies the placenta. This can help doctors make early diagnoses of conditions like high blood pressure, pregnancy toxaemia or pre-eclampsia.

A late scan

PREGNANCY STAGE
This may take place around 32 to 36 weeks of pregnancy.

PURPOSE
To check the position of the placenta and which way the baby is lying, to check that the baby is still growing properly and look for major physical defects.

There is no strong evidence that ultrasound scanning by itself carries any appreciable risk to the health of the fetus.

WHAT CAN BE SEEN
A final check can be made to see where the placenta is, and make an assessment of whether its position is going to cause any problems during a natural delivery.

At this stage of development the baby will be far too large to see much of him or her at any one time. Instead, the ultrasonographer will be able to make detailed examinations of individual areas and specific organs.

If there is any anxiety that the baby may not be growing as fast as he or she should, your midwife or doctor may ask you to go to the ultrasound clinic once a week so that the ultrasonographer can make regular measurements. This will help the healthcare team to give you the best advice.

This is also a good time to investigate any suspected heart problems or other physical abnormalities that will cause problems immediately after birth. By this stage, organs such as the kidneys and liver can be clearly seen and if the scan is continued for a long time you should be able to see the bladder filling and emptying.

Biochemical or hormonal markers

Another way of seeing how the baby is growing and developing is to measure the concentrations of various materials that are released from the baby into the mother's blood. These tests now form a major part of the antenatal screening programme.

The Alpha-fetoprotein (AFP) test

PREGNANCY STAGE

You may be invited to have a blood sample taken for this test between weeks 15 and 18.

PURPOSE

This was initially used on its own as a screening test for Down's syndrome or spina bifida. It gave results in terms of the chance of your baby having the condition, rather than an absolute yes or no. It is now almost always used only in combination with other tests.

RISKS

As the test is based on a sample of the mother's blood it poses no direct threat to the baby. However there is a distinct risk of causing unnecessary stress to the mother as the results are often not clear-cut. Many people end up with a 'false positive'—i.e. the test indicates the possibility of an abnormality when none is present. Because the test is imprecise you also run the risk of feeling you need to have further tests, such as an amniocentesis, which you may previously have ruled out because of the risk of it triggering a miscarriage.

WHAT IS INVOLVED

The test is performed on a sample of the mother's blood taken from her arm. It is designed to detect the amount of a specific protein, alpha-fetoprotein found in this blood sample (AFP is sometimes also called maternal serum alpha-fetoprotein MSAFP) .

Taking blood from the woman is considerably safer than taking samples from the unborn baby or its surroundings as in an amniocentesis. Unfortunately, the results are less accurate.

THE THEORY BEHIND THE TEST

AFP is produced in the liver and intestines of all growing babies. It is excreted into the amniotic fluid in the unborn baby's urine. The amniotic fluid is swallowed taking the AFP into the baby's gut from where it is absorbed into his or her bloodstream. Most of the AFP is broken down, but some passes across the placenta and into the mother's blood. A small amount of AFP can be measured in the mother's blood from the end of the third month of pregnancy and the concentration rises in the fourth and fifth months.

A higher than expected level of AFP could either indicate the presence of twins or that the pregnancy is more advanced than previously thought. However, it may also indicate that the baby has spina bifida (see page 88) or a severe head defect that is allowing AFP to flood into the amniotic fluid. On the other hand, lower than expected levels may indicate Down's syndrome. A detailed ultrasound scan may help to identify some of the causes of unusual AFP results and doctors may recommend that you go on to have an amniocentesis to check out the baby's chromosomes.

THE TEST RESULTS

You are very unlikely to be told the absolute values for the concentration of AFP in your blood. To a large degree that number is unimportant; it is the extent to which it is extreme for the age of the unborn baby that is of importance.

The problem is that used on its own this test is very inaccurate. Most mothers who have unusual levels of AFP in their blood are not carrying a baby with Down's syndrome or spina bifida. Conversely, just because the levels are normal does not mean that the baby is definitely not affected by either condition. Around 10 per cent of babies who have some abnormality are not detected by the test.

Bart's triple test

You may be invited to have a blood sample taken for this test from week 13 of pregnancy.

PURPOSE
This is a screening test specifically for Down's syndrome or spina bifida that gives a result in terms of the chance of your baby having the condition rather than an absolute yes or no.

RISKS
As for AFP testing.

WHAT IS INVOLVED
Owing to the uncertainty of interpreting the results of simply measuring AFP, doctors and scientists have developed tests that measure three substances in the woman's blood—AFP and two hormones, 'unconjugated oestriol' and 'human chorionic gonadotrophin'. The levels of these are used in conjunction with the woman's age to calculate her individual risk of having a baby with Down's syndrome. You should receive the results within seven to ten days of the blood sample being taken. The test got its name from the fact that it was developed at St Bartholomew's Hospital, London.

Some units offer a 'bivalent test' in which just two of these three hormones are monitored. They claim that the results are just as reliable as the triple test.

THE TEST RESULTS
It is important that the baby's age is known accurately, so that the results can be interpreted correctly. If there is doubt you may need an extra ultrasound scan so doctors can estimate the baby's age. This test detects around 60 per cent of babies with Down's syndrome. It therefore fails to detect just under half of the affected babies.

Also, you need to remember that once again the results only indicate an increased risk of the child having Down's syndrome; they do not say that the baby is definitely affected.

Bart's quadruple (or quad) test

PREGNANCY STAGE
You may be invited to have a blood sample taken for this test from 16 weeks of pregnancy.

PURPOSE
This is a screening test for Down's syndrome or spina bifida that gives a result in terms of the chance of your baby having the condition, rather than an absolute yes or no.

RISKS
As for AFP testing.

WHAT IS INVOLVED
As its name suggests, it measures four markers—the three used in the Bart's triple test, plus an additional type of human chorionic hormone. Once again, the results are used in conjunction with the woman's age to assess the probability of her child having Down's syndrome.

THE TEST RESULTS
This test has a detection rate of approximately 65 per cent.

Leeds triple plus test

PREGNANCY STAGE
You may be invited to have a blood sample taken for this test from 16 weeks of pregnancy.

PURPOSE
This is a screening test for Down's syndrome or spina bifida that gives a result in terms of the chance of your baby having the condition, rather than an absolute yes or no.

RISKS
As for AFP testing.

WHAT IS INVOLVED
This test is again based on a maternal blood sample, and measures AFP, human chorionic gonadotrophin and unconjugated oestriol. In addition, it measures the concentration of a compound called neutrophil alkaline phosphatase. One of the problems with this test is that neutrophil alkaline phosphatase breaks down quickly within the blood sample, so if it is not handled and stored correctly the results will be inaccurate. This lack of robustness has limited its use.

THE TEST RESULTS
The producers of the test claim that it will detect 85 per cent of babies with Down's syndrome, though not everyone agrees with this claim.

Maternal urine

Doctors and scientists are now turning to urine samples as part of their pursuit of ever safer and less invasive means of carrying out screening tests. They hope to be able to measure chemicals produced by the growing baby that may indicate a disability. These find their way into the mother's urine via her bloodstream.

The problem is that while this would provide a totally non-invasive method of testing it is likely to provide results that are less accurate. At the moment such tests are the preserve of research laboratories, but this means that before too long they will probably be added to the list of tests routinely offered.

Analysing some of the baby's cells

In the centre of each cell is a structure called a nucleus. This contains 46 chromosomes made of DNA. Written on these chromosomes are coded instructions, genes, that enable a person's body to be built and to function properly. Scientists estimate that there are some 100,000 genes and an error in the coding of just one of them can sometimes lead to a fatal or disabling disease. Owing to the way that a body grows, almost every cell in the body contains an identical set of genes.

By analysing a small sample of cells, you can find out whether the individual has the correct number of chromosomes, and whether they all look the right shape. Just because you have the right number of chromosomes does not mean you have a clean bill of health. There may still be minor errors in an individual chromosome that can cause a genetic disease. Some of these have been traced so that additional tests can confirm whether these faults are present or absent. However, it is not possible to look for every disease in every sample, so you will only be offered these tests if there is a history of a particular disease in your family.

Chorionic villus sampling (CVS)

PREGNANCY STAGE
The test sample is normally taken at 11 weeks of pregnancy.

PURPOSE
This is a method of collecting a small sample of cells that have been made by the growing baby. Consequently, they contain the same set of genetic information as is present in all of the baby's cells. Analysis of this sample gives clear answers about whether or not the baby has a chromosome abnormality, and can also identify specific genetic diseases.

Even in experienced hands, this technique carries a 1 in 50 to 1 in 100 risk of causing a miscarriage. Some centres report miscarriages of 5 per cent or more (1 in 20), and these should refer women to specialist centres, where the process is performed more frequently and with greater safety.

There is some anxiety that CVS may damage the unborn baby's limbs. At the moment there is insufficient evidence to prove this one way or the other. However, it appears that the main causes for concern are procedures carried out very early in pregnancy, around the eighth week. Doctors are consequently advising that CVS should not be used so early in pregnancy.

WHAT IS INVOLVED

An obstetrician uses a fine tube to take a sample of cells from the developing placenta. This tube is either passed through the woman's vagina and cervix, or via a needle which is inserted through her abdominal wall (see Figure 3). In either case, the tube is guided into position using an ultrasound scanner and collects a small sample of cells made by the growing baby. There is no evidence that one method is intrinsically better or safer than the other. The choice of sampling technique will be influenced largely by the way that the baby is lying and the location of the placenta. It will also be affected by local practice, as some centres become more used to performing one technique than the other and so prefer to use it whenever possible.

As the cells that make up the placenta are produced by the growing baby, they contain the same genetic information as the child. The chromosomes of these cells can be analysed in a laboratory and a variety of disorders, such as Down's syndrome and some genetic diseases, can be detected.

Doctors and midwives only recommend this procedure for women who already know that they have some increased risk of the baby having an abnormality. For example, the results of some

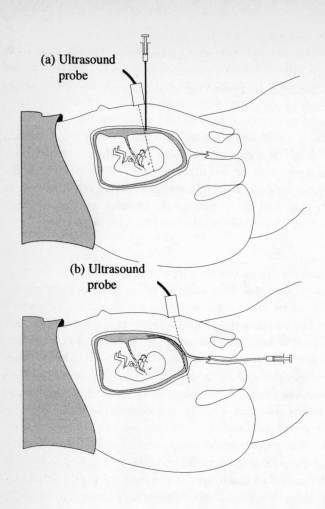

(a) Ultrasound
probe

(b) Ultrasound
probe

Figure 3: The two main methods used in chorionic villus sampling (CVS):
(a) the trans-abdominal method
(b) the trans-cervical method

other screening test have given cause for concern.

The name of the test comes from the fact that in early pregnancy doctors call the placenta the chorion and they remove the sample from an area of the chorion made up of finger-like projections called villi.

Amniocentesis

PREGNANCY STAGE
This procedure is normally carried out between 14 and 18 weeks of pregnancy.

PURPOSE
To collect a sample of the baby's cells from the amniotic fluid for the same laboratory analysis as with CVS tests.

RISKS
While the procedure should not disturb the unborn baby, it does carry a risk of causing a miscarriage, with about one in 200 babies miscarrying after the procedure. It is therefore only recommended for women over the age of 35 who are more likely to have a baby with Down's syndrome, or where there is a history of genetic disease in the family, or where a screening test has shown an increased risk.

There is also evidence that mid-term amniocentesis slightly increases the risk of the baby having respiratory problems once born. A possible explanation for this is that the procedure may disturb the growing baby just at the stage when the lungs are developing.

WHAT IS INVOLVED
The sample is taken by inserting a long syringe needle through the mother's abdominal wall into the amniotic sac (see Figure 4). Around 20 or 30 ml of fluid is drawn off and placed in sterile

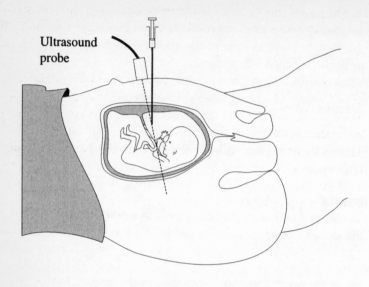

Ultrasound
probe

Figure 4: The method used in amniocentesis

pots. The mother may be given a local anaesthetic to minimize discomfort.

Amniotic fluid contains cells that have literally fallen off the baby or the tissues lining the inside of the sac in which the baby is growing. All of these cells contain the baby's chromosomes, because they have all grown from the fertilized egg.

THE TEST RESULTS

The results should be able to indicate whether the baby is male or female and also may tell you whether the baby has, or is carrying, specific genetic diseases. You should always discuss these results with a genetic counsellor, who will help you to understand their meaning.

Depending on the exact tests that are carried out, you may have to wait between 10 days and three weeks for the results.

Maternal blood

A tiny number of the baby's cells fall off the placenta and are carried away in the mother's bloodstream. Tests are being developed that can search for them and analyse their make-up. The major advantage in tests that look for cells in the mother's blood is that they should carry no risk of causing a miscarriage. At the moment these tests are confined to small research projects in major hospitals and it will probably be a number of years before any are brought into mainstream use.

Future possibilities

Experimental studies have been conducted that look for a protein called fetal fibronectin in the woman's vagina or cervix. Presence of this protein at around 24 to 27 weeks of pregnancy is a strong indicator of a premature labour.

There is also a suggestion that doctors should be screening for the presence of specific bacteria in the vagina, as these too may be responsible for triggering premature labour, which could kill the baby. If such bacteria are found, the infection could be abolished with a simple course of antibiotics.

Pre-implantation diagnosis of disease may be just around the corner. This is a technique that can only be used with methods of assisted reproduction, such as *in vitro* fertilization (IVF), where fertilization occurs in a laboratory. In this technique, a technician carefully removes one cell from an early embryo. Geneticists can then test this cell to see if the genes that it carries could cause particular diseases. By mid-1997, the procedure had been carried out at less than 10 centres around the world, and fewer than 50 babies had been born after being exposed to pre-implantation tests.

Additional problems for women of ethnic minorities

It is worth noting at this point that for many of the tests described here the results are more difficult to interpret for mothers-to-be from ethnic minorities. This is because doctors are increasingly realizing that the values chosen to indicate a healthy situation vary between ethnic groups, and insufficient work has been done to establish what is normal for many ethnic groups.

The standard tables used to draw conclusions from AFP and Leeds triple tests are based largely on studies of white-European or white-American populations. However, some laboratories have reported that the healthy AFP scores for members of Asian populations may be significantly higher than those found in the white populations. On top of this, the AFP scores for black populations can be as much as 22 per cent higher than the average for whites. Other laboratories have found similar differences in the values of human gonadotrophin, another one of the three chemicals measured in the Leeds triple and Bart's quad tests. They have discovered that women from Indian Asian groups have significantly higher levels of the hormone. If these differences are not taken into account then there is the real danger of faulty advice being given as women are incorrectly told that their baby is in a high-risk group for Down's syndrome. As a result, amniocentesis may be offered to people who really did not need it, thus exposing their baby to the risk of a miscarriage.

The problem is not just limited to measuring biochemical markers. Doctors use measurements of parts of the growing baby to assess whether he or she is growing properly. These measurements are made during routine ultrasound examinations. Once again, the normal values have been defined by studying whole populations that largely contain white Europeans or Americans. These people groups have a tendency to be physically larger than many other ethnic groups. As a result, the unborn baby of Asian parents may be incorrectly placed in a 'poor growth' group because he or she appears to be small according to the standard growth charts. Conversely, the excess growth in babies of ethnic women with diabetes may be missed. Sadly, very little is being done to address this situation—no one is sure what to do about it—but people from minority ethnic groups need to be warned.

Rosie

As Christians, Anne and Lindsey's first reaction to the scan, which showed that their baby was going to have severe deformities, was that they must continue the pregnancy whatever the outcome. After much heart-searching they changed their mind. They still consider that baby Rosie is part of their family's story.

'*I felt optimistic this time. Over the previous 12 months I had had two miscarriages, but this one had to be "third time lucky". An early scan confirmed my optimism and I could see a healthy heartbeat. But then a routine scan at 20 weeks dashed all my hopes. I was taken into the consultant's office and given the devastating news that our baby was severely deformed—no right leg at all, the left leg severely shortened and the right arm ended at the elbow. Only the left arm was unharmed. I was given the options available—termination, or full support if I decided to continue.*

'*My first reaction as a Christian was to say that we should continue. I had always thought that if a baby was alive, who was I to take that life away? But it is so easy to have strong principles when they are not being put to the test.*

'*Later at home, my husband and I discussed the problem at*

length. I found myself praying to have a miscarriage, when I had spent the previous 20 weeks praying not to. It was then that I realized what the right decision was for us. I just didn't want the responsibility of being the one to make it.

'The next morning, I visited our local vicar. He told me that sometimes it's not a case of a right decision, only a decision to be made for the right reasons. He was a wonderful comfort to me.

'We went to the hospital that afternoon and I was induced the following morning. I was left on my own in the gynae ward for the majority of the labour, which I later discovered had been very upsetting for the other patients on the ward. Many had been in tears for much of the day. I think it would have been better if I had been taken over to the labour ward much earlier.

'The consultant had promised me that there would be no need to endure pain, but this didn't prove to be the case. Sometimes, I felt that I couldn't bear the pain any longer and was eventually put on a morphine drip. It didn't ease the pain—I just seemed to float in and out of consciousness as each contraction hit.

'Our daughter Rosie was born just after 9 pm. They gave her to us and I was almost afraid to look. I had imagined a grotesquely deformed body, but she looked so beautiful. I know I looked at her limbs, but I can barely remember them, just the beautiful face. It was like looking in a mirror, because she looked just like me.

'They took her away to take photographs and then brought her back in a small Moses basket, dressed in a woollen hat and covered with a blanket. One of my biggest regrets is that she was photographed like this with only her face showing, as though the deformities had to be hidden. I would rather have a photo of her as she was, showing her misformed limbs.

'We held a private service at our local church and she was buried in the garden of remembrance. I don't visit the grave because Rosie isn't there, she's in our hearts and with us forever.

'The next few months were hard. In addition to the pain of losing a child, I felt a failure as a woman. After all, having babies was something any woman could do, wasn't it? Anyone but me, it seemed.

'The hospital staff gave me a copy of the SATFA handbook—I'm so glad they did. First it warned me that my milk would come in as my body didn't realize that my baby was dead. Secondly, it gave me a number to ring where I knew I wouldn't be told to 'pull yourself together'. Friends were very sympathetic, but seemed to expect me to be back to normal in a few weeks. It doesn't work like that.

'On the day that Rosie was supposed to be due, one of my best friends gave birth to a girl. It hurt so much. I was asked to be her godmother and as I held her it seemed to help. It also had the effect of making me want to try again.

'A month later I was pregnant with another baby. I was so scared. I was frightened that I wouldn't be able to love this baby because he or she wasn't Rosie. Edward was born a month premature and I loved him instantly.

'One morning when he was about three months old I woke up and realized that it was all over. I could parcel up the previous 20 months and call it a period in my life. I have a wonderful husband, a beautiful son, a lovely new house and life was more than just worth living again. I was happy. We'll never forget Rosie, and it still makes me sad sometimes, but the pain has gone.'

7

Specific diseases

Specific diseases can be grouped under chromosomal (gross damage to whole chromosomes), genetic (faulty single genes), or congenital (diseases that you are born with, but have not necessarily been inherited from either parent) abnormalities. The common diseases are listed along with their cause; the frequency in the population; any characteristic symptoms; an indication of the effect on the person's life and a list of the tests used during pregnancy to detect the condition.

Chromosomal abnormalities

In the relatively few years that have followed the discovery of DNA, there has been an explosion in our knowledge and understanding of genetics. DNA is the chemical used by almost all living cells to file all the information needed to build our bodies. This DNA is contained in chromosomes that are found within the cell's nucleus. These chromosomes are chain-like structures, with a unit of DNA making up each of the links. Each link in the chain is effectively one 'letter' of a code which contains the cell's working instructions. The code is divided into discrete sections called genes. Human beings are thought to have a total of some 100,000 genes 'written', using over 3,000 million letters.

Most people have 46 chromosomes in each often thought of as belonging to two sets. First, th of chromosomes carrying genes that regulate functions, the autosomal chromosomes. Secon further two chromosomes that, as well as instructions, have the additional task of establishing the sex of the individual. In females both of these two will be X chromosomes, and in males there will be one X and one Y. Not surprisingly, the X and Y chromosomes are called the sex chromosomes.

The reason why you look a bit like your mother and a bit like your father is that when an egg and sperm fuse together they each bring one of each autosome and one sex chromosome. With 23 chromosomes from each parent, the new individual sets out in life with a full complement of 46.

The egg will always carry an X chromosome, but the man's sperm carries either an X or a Y chromosome. If an egg is fertilized by a sperm bearing an X chromosome, then the new individual will be female. If it is fertilized by a sperm containing a Y chromosome, then a male will result.

So far so good. However, in a few cases a person starts life with an extra copy of one chromosome, or significant damage to a chromosome. In most cases the result is that no development occurs and no one knows anything about it. Occasionally the baby starts to grow, but dies early on, leading to a miscarriage. But there are instances where extra or damaged chromosomes are tolerated and the baby survives with a set of symptoms that are characteristic of that particular chromosomal abnormality. Down's syndrome is one of the best-known examples. Although we can count the number of chromosomes, the reason why some people appear to be severely affected and others only mildly affected is unknown.

There appear to be two basic routes by which the person acquires the extra chromosome. The most common one is where two copies of the chromosome manage to get into either the egg or the sperm during their production.

...ess common cause is where part of a chromosome has ...ken off and joined onto the end of another chromosome. This may occur in either parent and is called a chromosome translocation. The parent is unaffected by this, and when an egg or sperm forms there may be the correct number of chromosomes, but too many copies of the genes found on that chromosome. The consequence of this is that there are families who are at a high risk of having children with specific syndromes. If you are a member of such a family, you may wish to have a chromosome analysis to see if your offspring are likely to be affected.

Down's syndrome

CAUSE

Only in 1959 did doctors discover that the cause of Down's syndrome was an extra chromosome. Those affected have three copies of chromosome 21 instead of two, so the condition is sometimes called trisomy 21. For some reason, this disturbance of the balance leads to the condition.

The chance of a woman producing an egg containing two chromosome 21s seems to increase with age, to the point that there is a noticeable increase in risk once a woman is over 35, indicating that the defect more often occurs during egg rather than sperm production.

INCIDENCE

In the UK, about 1 in 1,000 babies born is affected by the syndrome. The risk is strongly affected by the mother's age. As women approach and pass the age of 35 their chance of having a baby with Down's syndrome increases markedly (see Figure 5). There is some evidence that the incidence of Down's syndrome may reduce in women over the age of 45. However, this is probably due to the small amount of data available in this age group, as very few women of that age get pregnant.

Like everyone, people with Down's syndrome have many characteristics that they inherit from their family. In addition, they have a group of distinctive physical characteristics, as well as learning difficulties. Most people with the syndrome have eyes that slope down towards the nose, a large tongue, and hands that tend to be short and broad. The extent to which these characteristics are evident varies between individuals.

Around 40 per cent of these children are also born with heart defects which may or may not require surgery. They can also have difficulty with hearing, vision, and some have intestinal problems.

OUTLOOK

Many people with Down's syndrome grow up to be capable of living semi-independent lives, and are capable of reading and writing, while others will need more support throughout their lives. Their IQs tend to range between 30 and 80; most people's IQ ranges from 80 to 120.

According to the Down's Syndrome Association, at the beginning of the 20th century, the average life expectancy of people with Down's syndrome was less than 10 years. Now it is at least 60 years—a 655.5 per cent increase. As adults, they often have normal expectations of achievement and a desire to form close relationships.

As there are now more older people with Down's syndrome, a link between the syndrome and Alzheimer's disease has become apparent. The reason for this is believed to be connected with the fact that there is a genetic link between a gene on chromosome 21 and Alzheimer's disease, and people with Down's syndrome have an extra copy of this chromosome. Recent research shows that a very small percentage of people with Down's syndrome develop dementia between the ages of 30 and 39. By the age of 49 this increases to 10 per cent and is up

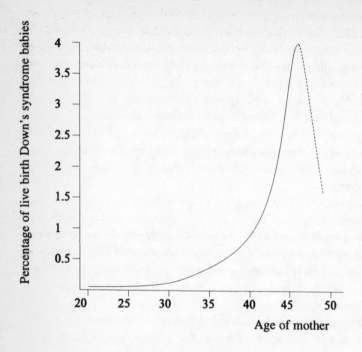

Figure 5: This graph shows the percentage chance of a woman of a particular age giving birth to a live baby with Down's syndrome.

to 40 per cent by the age of 60. Even though these figures show that some people with the syndrome will develop dementia, they also show that the majority won't. To put these figures into context, it is unusual for an otherwise healthy person to develop dementia before they are 60 years old.

PRENATAL DIAGNOSIS

AFP, triple or quad blood screening tests are used to indicate the chance that a baby may have Down's syndrome. Ultrasound scanning early in pregnancy, often called the King's Down's syndrome screening test or nuchal fold scan, can also give an indication. Collecting samples of cells that contain the baby's genetic material either by CVS or amniocentesis can almost always confirm whether or not the syndrome is present.

Edward's syndrome

CAUSE
Three copies of chromosome 18 (Trisomy 18).

INCIDENCE
Approximately 1 in 3,000. More girls are born with the syndrome than boys, but this is probably because boys with this chromosomal abnormality have a greater tendency to die during pregnancy, or miscarry. As in Down's syndrome the incidence increases as the mother gets older.

SYMPTOMS
Multiple abnormalities. Consult a genetic counsellor.

OUTLOOK
Three out of 10 babies die within the first month after birth. Those surviving more than a year have severely delayed development.

PRENATAL DIAGNOSIS
CVS or amniocentesis can be used to find out if there is an incorrect number of chromosomes in the baby's cells, and would only be recommended where there is a history of the disease in the family, or when the mother is over 35 years old.

Patau syndrome

CAUSE
Three copies of chromosome 13 (Trisomy 13).

INCIDENCE
Approximately 1 in 5,000. Once again, the incidence increases as the mother gets older.

SYMPTOMS
Multiple malformations, including heart disease and cleft palate.

OUTLOOK
Nine out of 10 die before they reach one year old.

PRENATAL DIAGNOSIS
CVS or amniocentesis can be used to find out if there is an incorrect number of chromosomes in the baby's cells, and would only be recommended where there is a history of the disease in the family.

47, XXY (Klinefelter's syndrome)

CAUSE
There are two possible causes:
1. The X chromosomes in the egg fail to separate properly, so that the egg contains two copies. When this combines with a Y-carrying sperm the result is a *male* embryo with one too many X chromosomes.
2. The X and Y chromosomes in the sperm fail to separate, so the sperm contributes both an X and a Y and the egg contributes another X.

Overall, the incidence is about 1 in 1,000 births, but there is an increased risk as the mother gets older.

SYMPTOMS
These individuals have poorly developed secondary sexual characteristics and they are usually infertile. Most of them have only slightly reduced verbal and mental skills, though a few will be more severely affected. There is a tendency for them to be quite tall.

OUTLOOK
Day-to-day living may hardly be affected, but some do have learning difficulties and need the help of a special school.

PRENATAL DIAGNOSIS
This can be detected by counting the number of chromosomes in the baby's cells, collected by either amniocentesis or CVS.

47, XXX

CAUSE
There are two possible causes:

1. The X chromosomes in the egg fail to separate properly, so that the egg contains two copies. When this combines with an X-carrying sperm, the result is a female embryo with one too many X chromosomes.

2. The X and Y chromosomes in the cells that form sperm separate, and then the X chromosome replicates. This allows the sperm to contribute two X chromosomes to the embryo.

INCIDENCE
Overall, the incidence is about 1 in 1,000 births, but it increases as the mother gets older.

Individuals may have slight learning difficulties, though otherwise they are clinically normal (i.e. they look and behave like any other healthy child). Sexual development and fertility is unaffected and is therefore normal.

OUTLOOK
Day-to-day living may hardly be affected but some do have learning difficulties and need the help of a special school.

PRENATAL DIAGNOSIS
This can be detected by counting the number of chromosomes in cells collected by either amniocentesis or CVS.

45, X (Turner's syndrome)

CAUSE
This results when either the sperm carries no X or Y chromosome, or the egg has no X chromosome.

INCIDENCE
One in 10,000 births

SYMPTOMS
The necks of people with Turner's syndrome have thick 'webbing', and they tend to be short of stature. They have normal intelligence, but puberty may be delayed. Some also have heart defects.

OUTLOOK
People with this condition have normal life spans.

PRENATAL DIAGNOSIS
The thickened neck may be discovered at an early nuchal ultrasound scan. The condition is then almost always confirmed by amniocentesis or CVS.

Genetic abnormalities

There is no way that this chapter can unpack the full story of genetic disease. However, it will outline the basic principles involved, so that you are in a better position to ask appropriate questions when you talk with any health professional.

Genetic abnormalities occur when the genetic code contains a spelling mistake that disrupts one or more genes. The damaged gene fails to perform properly and, as a consequence, a particular function is lost, resulting in a 'genetic abnormality' or 'genetic disease'. A well-known example of this is cystic fibrosis, where a single letter spelling mistake in a single gene found on chromosome 7 can prevent cells building a specific protein. Without this protein, cells that need to secrete mucus cannot work and the person suffers from a variety of sometimes life-threatening symptoms.

The more scientists discover about genetics, the more complex the subject becomes. All the same, it is possible to divide the most common genetic diseases into a number of different types.

Single gene defects

In 1988, a list was published of 4,344 diseases which were believed to result from a single faulty gene. Hardly a week goes by without the location of one of these errant genes being pinpointed on one or other chromosome. Each time a gene is 'mapped' or located, it heralds the possibility of developing laboratory tests which can determine whether individual people have a healthy or unhealthy version of this particular gene. All you need to perform a test is a small sample of the person's cells. After birth they are easy to collect, either by wiping a swab around inside the mouth, or by taking a small blood sample. Before birth, you have the added complication of an amniocentesis or CVS.

Genetic mechanism	Resulting disease	Symptoms	Frequency per 10,000 births
Autosomal recessive	Cystic fibrosis	Thick mucus secretion—chest infections	5-6
	Phenylketonuria	Mental handicap	1
	Tays Sachs disease	Mental handicap and blindness	0.04
	Congenital deafness	Deaf from birth	5
Autosomal dominant	Huntington's disease	Involuntary movement and dementia from middle age	2
	Polycystic disease	Progressive kidney failure	10
	Otosclerosis	Reduced hearing from adolescence or later	30
Sex-linked	Haemophilia	Severe bleeding after injury	3
	Childhood blindness	Blindness	0.2
	Duchenne type muscular dystrophy	Progressive weakening of muscles leading to death, usually in the 30s	3

Table 5: Conditions caused by errors in single genes

There are various ways that an error in one of these genes may affect a person (see Table 5).

AUTOSOMAL RECESSIVE

As we established earlier, 44 of each cell's chromosomes occur in 22 pairs, the autosomes. That means that there are two copies of each gene, one on each member of the pair. In some situations, if one gene is faulty but its pair is fine, then the one healthy gene will win out and the person will not be affected. The unhealthy

Autosomal recessive condition

One parent is a carrier

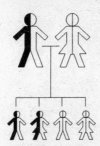

Regardless of sex,
1 in 2 are carriers

Both parents are carriers

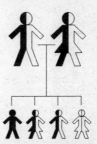

Regardless of sex,
1 in 4 are affected
1 in 2 are carriers

One parent is affected

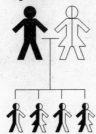

All are carriers

In a recessive condition carriers will be healthy

Figure 6: Inheritance pattern in autosomal recessive families

gene is said to be recessive. People only have symptoms of an autosomal recessive disease if they have two faulty copies.

People with one faulty and one healthy gene are called

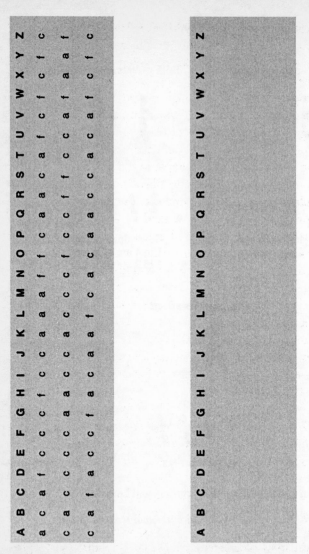

Table 6: Flicking coins 2. On this occasion I ended up with one family where every child was affected by the condition, three families where all the children were carriers, and one family where every child was free of the disease-causing gene. However, looking at the total population 25 were affected (a), 36 were carriers (c) and 17 were free (f). This is close to the 1 : 2 : 1 ratio that we would expect.

carriers. This is because, although they are not affected, they can pass the gene on to their offspring (see Figure 6). If the offspring receives a second faulty gene from the other parent, then he or she may have the disease.

The passage of this gene through the population follows the general principles of chance. If you can discover how many people carry a single defective gene then you can soon calculate how many people are likely to be affected by the condition. For example, we know that 1 in 25 people in the UK carries a single faulty copy of the gene for cystic fibrosis. Now, because the disease results from a recessive gene (i.e. the disease will appear in the offspring only when not masked by a dominant healthy gene), a person will not be affected unless he or she carries two faulty copies of the gene, one on each of the chromosome pair. For this to occur, both of his or her parents must carry at least one faulty copy. The chance of both parents carrying a single copy of the gene is 1 in 625 (i.e. 1 in 25 multiplied by 1 in 25). Even if both parents carry a single copy of the gene there is only a 1 in 4 chance of one of their offspring inheriting both parents' faulty genes and consequently being affected by the disease. Therefore we arrive at the average risk for an individual member of the population of 1 in 2,500 (i.e. 1 in 4 multiplied by 1 in 625). This is indeed the rate at which cystic fibrosis occurs naturally. The occurrence of the disease is being reduced, as affected families use this knowledge to influence their decisions about having children.

So, what is the risk of a couple having one or more children affected by a genetic disease, if they know that they are carriers of a faulty gene? Let's go back to our coins.

This time you need two coins so that we can have a look at how the principles of chance affect a family with a history of genetic disease. For simplicity, let's choose a situation where in each family both the mother and the father have one healthy gene and one unhealthy disease-causing gene (i.e. both parents are carriers). If the child inherits two unhealthy genes, one from each parent, he will be affected by the condition. If he inherits only one copy then he is a carrier, but is healthy, and if he inherits no unhealthy gene then he is free of the condition—neither affected by the condition, nor a carrier of it.

Get a fresh piece of paper. Mark out your grid again (see Table 6) and this time flick both coins at the same time. If both come up tails, mark the child as being affected by the condition—'A'. If one heads and one tails, then mark the child 'C'—a carrier. If both are heads mark down 'F'—for free from the condition. Work all the way along the 26 families giving each family three children. You are almost bound to find that for some families life is 'unfair'—they have had three affected offspring. Other families have had a clear run of unaffected children. If you count up all of the As, Cs and Fs you will find that they are in a ratio very close to 1:2:1—that is, there will be around 20 As, 20 Fs and around 40 Cs.

There is nothing magical about the process. It is all due to the way that chance works.

AUTOSOMAL DOMINANT
Other diseases occur if either member of a gene pair has a fault. The diseased gene appears to dominate over the healthy copy. Therefore, if you have one healthy and one affected gene you will be affected by the disease. The pattern of inheritance is more straightforward. If either parent has one of these errant genes, there is a 1 in 2 chance that the offspring will inherit the gene and be affected by the condition (see Figure 7).

SEX-LINKED
In both of the above cases, the disease is as likely to affect males as it is to affect females. A third set of conditions exists, in which the faulty genes are located only on the X chromosome. Now, females carry two X chromosomes, but men only have one.

Autosomal dominant conditions

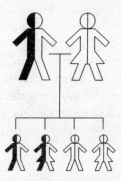

**Regardless of sex,
1 in 2 are affected**

*Figure 7: Inheritance pattern in autosomal dominant families.
One parent is affected—the half-shading shows that the father has only
one diseased gene, but because the disease is dominant he still has the
disease.*

Where the disease is recessive, a woman who has one faulty gene
and one healthy copy will be all right because the healthy gene
will always dominate. Women, then, only have problems if both
copies of this gene are damaged. However, as males only have
one X chromosome, if it carries a faulty gene, it will cause a
disease. The result is that on the whole women can act as
carriers, while men suffer from the condition.

If the father carries an affected X chromosome and both the
mother's X chromosomes are free of the disease, all boys receive
their one X chromosome from their mother and are therefore
unaffected. However, all girls receive one healthy X chromosome

from their mother and one affected chromosome from their father—they are therefore carriers. If, on the other hand, it is the mother who carries a single affected X chromosome then there is a 50 per cent chance that they will receive a disease-bearing copy. Therefore, 1 in 2 sons will be affected and 1 in 2 daughters will be carriers (see Figure 8).

Sex-linked conditions

Father is affected	Mother is a carrier

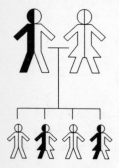 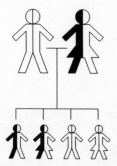

All sons are unaffected
All daughters are carriers

1 in 2 sons are affected
1 in 2 daughters are carriers

Figure 8: Inheritance pattern in sex-linked disease

Probably the most famous example of this type of inheritance is the pattern of haemophilia within the royal families of Europe. With the benefit of hindsight, gained by looking at a family tree, it is easy to see which women carried the disease and unwittingly passed it on to the next generation. It is most likely that the disease started as a spontaneous mutation in the reproductive cells of Queen Victoria or one of her parents (see Figure 9).

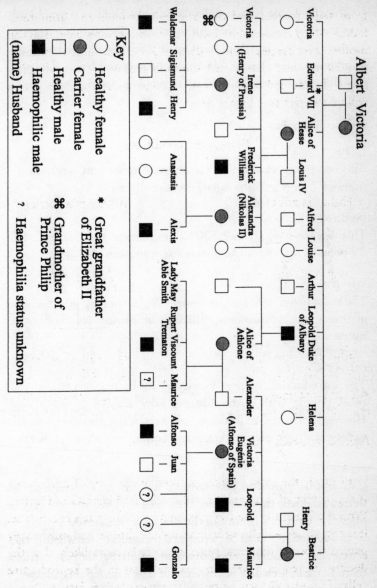

Figure 9: Queen Victoria's legacy of haemophilia

123

The effect that haemophilia had on the families is graphically displayed by the fact that Alfonso and Gonzalo, the sons of Victoria Eugenie and Alfonso of Spain, accidentally bled to death. In addition, Henry, son of Henry of Prussia and Irene, died aged 4—although his brother Waldemar survived until he was 56.

Cystic fibrosis

CAUSE
This condition is caused by a faulty gene located on chromosome number 7. It is an autosomal recessive disease.

INCIDENCE
This disease affects 1 in 2,500 babies born in the UK, with 1 in 25 people carrying single affected chromosomes.

SYMPTOMS
The most prominent symptoms are long-term lung infections. In addition, the person has difficulty absorbing fats and other nutrients.

OUTLOOK
The introduction of new ranges of antibiotics has meant that most people with cystic fibrosis now survive to adulthood. However, affected individuals will need daily treatment with a variety of drugs, physiotherapy and sometimes a special diet.

PRENATAL DIAGNOSIS
CVS is usually used to take samples for genetic analysis that can detect whether the baby has the disease. This would only be offered if there is a history of the disease in the family.

In addition, tests can be performed on adults to see whether they are carriers. If both members of a couple find that they are carriers, there is a 1 in 4 chance of any child of theirs having the disease.

There is some debate about launching a national screening

programme to identify carriers of this gene. The application of such a programme will need careful ethical consideration.

Haemophilia

CAUSE
X-linked recessive disease, although spontaneous mutations do occur.

INCIDENCE
Approximately 1 in 5,000 males.

SYMPTOMS
This is a disorder in which the person does not manufacture enough of a compound called factor VIII. This factor is needed to help blood clot in a wound. Without it, they bleed profusely if injured. Bleeding often occurs inside joints, causing swelling, pain and disability.

Some people are severely affected by the disease, while others have only mild symptoms. Those with the condition need to inject factor VIII each time they have an injury.

OUTLOOK
Children with haemophilia need to be encouraged to participate in non-contact sports such as swimming, because games like football or rugby will cause massive internal bleeding. A bump that would cause a tiny bruise for most people could be life-threatening for someone with haemophilia. The long-term outlook varies enormously between individuals, as some die in early childhood and others live full and fulfilled lives.

CVS or amniocentesis can be used to look for a damaged gene if a family history of the disease is already identified. Also, in affected families, determining the sex of the baby can be useful, as all girls are safe from being affected themselves, although they may be carriers of the disease.

Female relatives of people with haemophilia may want to seek genetic counselling before starting a family, as they may be carrying an affected gene.

There are moves at some major centres for fertility treatment to introduce pre-implantation sex-selection. In this procedure, technicians can determine the sex of embryos created in a laboratory. The carriers of haemophilia will be able to choose to implant only female embryos. The children will be their natural genetic children, just conceived using the techniques of *in vitro* fertilization (IVF).

Fragile X

CAUSE

This is caused by a genetic error in the X chromosome, that causes sections of that chromosome to be missing. Women may carry the disease and pass it on to male offspring.

INCIDENCE

Approximately 1 in 2,000 male births. Some 1 in 1,000 women are carriers of, or mildly affected by, the disease. This is the greatest genetic cause of learning difficulty, after Down's syndrome.

SYMPTOMS

Moderate or severe mental retardation. Affected males are often tall and strong with a prominent jaw and nose. They have increased ear length, over-large testes and are prone to epileptic seizures.

One third of the females who are carriers of the disease have mild learning difficulties.

OUTLOOK
People with fragile X have a normal life expectancy.

PRENATAL DIAGNOSIS
Where there is a family history of the disease, CVS or amniocentesis can give an indication of whether the baby is affected.

Phenylketonuria (PKU)

CAUSE
Autosomal recessive.

INCIDENCE
One in 16,000 babies (1 in 7,500 in Scotland).

SYMPTOMS
If the condition is not detected, infants will start to have epilepsy and will develop severe learning difficulties. Affected children also tend to be affected by eczema.

OUTLOOK
If detected, and the child is placed on a diet that is low in the amino acid phenylalanine, then he or she has every chance for normal growth and development and a healthy life span.

PRENATAL DIAGNOSIS
Amniocentesis or CVS can be offered to pregnant women whose families are affected by the condition. After birth, it is detected by a routine blood sample taken by a midwife from the baby's heel.

Sickle cell disease

CAUSE
Autosomal recessive.

INCIDENCE
One in 200 people of West Indian ethnic origin are affected, along with 1 in 100 people of West African ethnic origin and 1 in 4 people who live in or originate from Nigeria. As a result 1 in 10 Black people living in the UK carry a single copy of the gene.

SYMPTOMS
The red blood cells of affected people contain an unusual protein, which causes the cells to buckle into a sickle or 'S' shape. The cells are fragile and break up. They also have difficulty passing through small blood vessels inside organs. The net result is a long-term and severe form of anaemia. This results in fatigue, headaches and jaundice. Children with the disease are particularly prone to poisoning and pneumonia.

OUTLOOK
Some affected individuals have only mild symptoms, but in others the symptoms are severe and disabling.

PRENATAL DIAGNOSIS
CVS, amniocentesis or direct analysis of a blood sample taken from the baby after 13 weeks of pregnancy can be used to detect the disease. You can also test parents to see if they are carrying the disease and have the ability to pass it on to their offspring. Afro-Caribbean people are routinely tested at antenatal clinics.

Thalassaemia

CAUSE

This is an autosomal recessive disease. The genetic fault causes an imbalance in the proportion of two different forms of haemoglobin—the material that carries oxygen around our bodies in red blood cells. Healthy individuals have equal quantities of alpha and beta haemoglobin. In people with thalassaemia, the ratio is unbalanced and the blood cells become fragile. The end result is a form of anaemia.

In alpha-thalassaemia the production of alpha chains is disrupted; in beta-thalassaemia the production of beta chains is disrupted.

INCIDENCE

Members of the Mediterranean, Middle Eastern and South-East Asian ethnic populations are most at risk from thalassaemia. Of the Europeans, 1 in 6 Cypriots, 1 in 14 Greeks and 1 in 50 Italians carry the affected genes.

Beta-thalassaemia is the more common form of the disease. If a person inherits one gene, they will have a mild form of the disease—known as beta-thalassaemia minor—which is never severe. Inheriting two copies of the faulty gene causes a severe version of the disease called beta-thalassaemia major. Alpha-thalassaemia is much less common.

SYMPTOMS AND OUTLOOK

Beta-thalassaemia major causes anaemia, jaundice, fatigue and breathlessness. The symptoms appear within a few months of birth. Without treatment the person will die early in childhood, but now, with repeated transfusions, the majority survive.

Beta-thalassaemia minor causes only mild symptoms and leaves the person free to live a normal life.

Alpha-thalassaemia spans a range of symptoms and outlook. At one extreme it can be so severe that the child dies within a few hours of birth. At the other extreme it causes a mild form of anaemia.

Passing a long needle through the mother's tummy to take a blood sample directly from the unborn baby's umbilical cord allows analysis and detection of the disease. If an exact mutation is already known within the family, then examination of cells collected by CVS or amniocentesis can also indicate whether or not the child is affected.

Tay-Sachs

CAUSE
Recessive autosomal disease that prevents a particular enzyme, hexosaminidase A, being formed.

INCIDENCE
Tay-Sachs disease is most common in Jewish ethnic populations, and in particular the Ashkenazi Jews, where it affects 1 in 2,500 people, with 1 in 25 members of this ethnic group being a carrier. This is 100 times higher than for other members of the population.

SYMPTOMS
A rare but fatal neurological disease that first appears within six months of birth. The initial signs of blindness are rapidly followed by dementia, seizure and paralysis.

OUTLOOK
Affected children usually die before the age of four.

PRENATAL DIAGNOSIS
Analysis of cells collected by CVS or amniocentesis is possible. The orthodox Jewish community around the world has established a

confidential screening system to help people select marriage partners. Everyone has a test and is given a reference number but not told the result. When two people are considering getting married, they submit the two reference numbers. If both people are carrying the defective gene they are warned. If only one or neither has the gene they are informed that any children they may conceive in the future are safe from the effects of this particular disease. There is always the possibility that one of them may be a carrier and, if so, their children may also end up being carriers.

Other Jewish people are tested at open sessions arranged by their community or request testing through the antenatal clinic.

Multifactorial conditions

So far, we have only considered genetic abnormalities where a single faulty gene causes a clearly recognizable set of symptoms. However, many diseases or abnormalities only occur if there is damage to more than one gene. In addition, they often require a particular set of environmental circumstances to trigger the symptoms. Such multifactorial conditions are much more difficult to monitor and predict.

The theory is that many different genes regulate the healthy function that normally prevents these diseases. If a few of the genes are faulty then the body manages to cope, but if too many are damaged then the symptoms appear.

Conditions such as cleft lip and palate, congenital dislocation of hips, insulin-dependent diabetes and insulin-independent diabetes have all been identified as multifactorial diseases. For a couple who have had one child with a congenital malformation, the risk of this being repeated in subsequent children is between 2 and 5 per cent.

Gene therapy

How about the possibility of giving a healthy copy of the gene to someone who has a disease resulting from a faulty gene? This is the realm of gene therapy.

For a few months in the spring of 1993 the media were full of the hope that genetic therapy was about to cure previously untreatable diseases. A young child by the name of Carly Todd had been given a treatment that effectively introduced a healthy copy of a particular gene into the cells that manufacture her blood cells. Her own copy of this gene was defective and, as a result, she was incapable of fighting infections.

At the time, the scientists and doctors involved knew that the chances of success were slim, and indeed it now appears that the new gene did not become established. She continues to suffer from the disease, which leaves her with little or no immune system.

A few other attempts at similar treatments have been made in the US with little more success and, at the moment, scientific commentators are viewing the whole area with increased caution.

Congenital abnormalities

Heart defects

CAUSE
The cause of over half of heart defects is unknown. In these cases there is a 2 to 3 per cent chance of subsequent children having the same problem. One third are the result of some known genetic disease, and you will need to consult a genetic counsellor to discover the risk for any future children.

INCIDENCE
One in every 100 children have some heart abnormality.

Most are of no concern. If they are serious, blueish skin and breathlessness are the two key symptoms and they may first appear at any age. Occasionally, heart defects are not detected until adulthood.

OUTLOOK
A wide range of conditions can now be treated with drugs or surgery, with excellent results, though some remain life-threatening. Many, however, need no treatment at all.

PRENATAL DIAGNOSIS
Ultrasound scans may detect some major defects, often in association with other conditions, such as Down's syndrome.

Neural tube defects—spina bifida, anencephaly.

CAUSE
During development in the first few weeks after conception, cells migrate to precise locations and form new organs. Some form a tube-like structure that develops into the brain and spinal cord. In the embryo, this structure is called the neural tube, so if anything goes wrong with its development you get a neural tube defect (NTD).

In spina bifida, a failure causes the spinal cord to be left unprotected and vulnerable to damage. In anencephaly, a different failure prevents the formation of large parts of the brain.

INCIDENCE
Sixteen out of 1,000 babies conceived in the UK have some form of neural tube defect, although only 1 in 1,000 children born have one of these conditions. This is partly due to the number of spontaneous miscarriages and partly to prenatal screening followed by terminations.

In the UK, more children born during the winter are affected and there is a higher incidence in lower social classes.

The incidence of the disease is falling at a greater rate than can be explained by miscarriages and terminations and is probably explained by the fact that women's health and diet is improving. Having an adequate level of folic acid in the woman's diet is known to help prevent spina bifida in the majority (70 per cent) of families. For some as yet unknown reason, in the remaining 30 per cent of families folic acid appears to give no protection. Green vegetables are a good source of this nutrient, but to avoid running the risk of having a low intake, doctors recommend that women supplement their natural intake with a tablet containing 400 µg (micrograms) of folic acid per day from a month before they get pregnant and then for the first three months of pregnancy. (As many pregnancies start without planning, the woman should start the supplement as soon as she realizes the situation.)

If you have had one child with a neural tube defect the chance of having a second affected child is 1 in 30. However, this can be reduced to 1 in 70 by taking a high-dose supple ment of 5 mg of folic acid each day.

SYMPTOMS AND OUTLOOK
People with spina bifida vary enormously in their symptoms. Around a quarter have little or no disability, while others have some degree of paralysis in their arms and legs. Some babies will require surgery within 24 hours of birth if they are going to have a reasonable chance of survival.

Children with anencephaly often die during pregnancy, leading to a miscarriage. Those that survive to birth seldom live for more than a few days.

PRENATAL DIAGNOSIS
Prenatal AFP blood tests give an indication of the possibility of a problem (i.e. there is a high false-positive rate). This can often, but not always, be confirmed with a detailed ultrasound scan.

Hydrocephalus

CAUSE
The problem is sometimes associated with a neural tube defect, a viral defect or, occasionally, a rare genetic defect.

INCIDENCE
One in 1,000 births is affected.

SYMPTOMS
In hydrocephalus, the movement of fluid (cerebrospinal fluid) inside the baby's brain is blocked. The fluid collects over the brain leading to an increase in the pressure within the skull. For this reason it is often known as 'water on the brain'. This, in turn, causes the head to swell and also prevents the brain from developing. The exact reason why the fluid build-up occurs is often unknown.

OUTLOOK
In severe cases of hydrocephalus the baby will die at or shortly after birth. However, with early diagnosis and treatment the long-term outlook for less severe cases can be reasonable. But often the situation is not detected until some brain damage has occurred.

PRENATAL DIAGNOSIS
A mid-term ultrasound scan can usually detect this problem as the baby develops.

Umbilical hernia (exomphalos)

CAUSE
The reason why this occurs is often unknown, though sometimes it is due to a chromosomal abnormality.

INCIDENCE
One in 1,000 births is affected.

SYMPTOMS

The wall of the tummy has a defect and either one or two loops of the baby's gut, or the whole gut and stomach, develop outside the baby in the amniotic fluid.

OUTLOOK

If the baby's chromosomes are normal then surgical repair after birth is usually successful and the child should live a normal life. In about a third of these cases such hernias are associated with serious genetic or chromosomal abnormalities. Then the outlook may not be so good.

PRENATAL DIAGNOSIS

This is normally detected at the mid-pregnancy ultrasound scan. At that stage it can look more frightening than it really is.

Harriet

Harriet hadn't given the tests a second thought when she became pregnant for the first time. Now pregnant with her second child, she is adamant that she would not take the AFP test.

'I'm 31 years old and expecting my second child. However, when I was pregnant with my first child I had the AFP and about two weeks later I got a call from the advice nurse who said that, based on the test, I had a 1 in 120 chance of having a baby with Down's syndrome. I was in such shock that I didn't really know what questions to ask. She tried to calm me down, saying that my test was most likely indicating a "false positive", but that the only way to be certain was to have an amniocentesis. She offered to set up an appointment with a genetics counsellor and asked if I was interested in having the amniocentesis. I numbly replied: "Yes". At this point, I didn't think to ask for a retest, or ask for more detailed information.

'I suppose that it is one thing for the medical staff to do their best to help you to be as relaxed as possible, but when my husband called her back the day before our appointment with the geneticist, to ask questions, she was quite nonchalant! Very disturbing!

'We saw the genetics counsellor, who explained the risks of Down's syndrome for the average woman my age, and my risk as indicated by the test. I was immediately suspicious when she explained that the dates used in testing were based on the timing of my last menstrual period. I felt that my "real" dates differed slightly from the dates in my medical notes, so the geneticist reran the calculations. By moving the dates only half of one week, the risk changed from 1 in 120 to only 1 in 200; and they consider anything better than 1 in 200 normal.

'So, rather than an amniocentesis, we had a detailed ultrasound examination. From this, the doctors were able to confirm the dates of my last menstrual period to within a week—this is the best that you can get with ultrasound. But this was no better than we knew already, so the doctor couldn't change the date used to calculate my risk. Luckily, there were no indications of Down's syndrome from the ultrasound.

'My husband felt reassured that nothing was wrong, but I was now so disturbed that I really needed to be certain. So, in the end we also opted for the amniocentesis. Amazingly, we found out the results in only a week (rather than the two to three weeks the advice nurse had originally told us). Our baby girl does not have Down's syndrome.

'With my second baby, I have no intention of putting myself through all that again. The anguish we went through was horrible and we were really lucky not to have to wait so long for the results of the amniocentesis. The AFP is so imprecise that half a week meant all the difference in terms of dating the pregnancy. I'm not surprised that it commonly gives false positives. This time around I'd much rather have a detailed ultrasound and simply skip the AFP.'

Notes
1. *Mendelian Inheritance in Man*, by Victor McKusick (8th edition, John Hopkins University Press, Baltimore, MD, USA).

8

Operating on babies before birth

In a few cases doctors can detect problems that can be solved or made less severe by relatively simple operations performed while the baby is still in the womb.

In giving a window into the womb, ultrasound has opened the possibility not only of observing potential problems, but also of treating them. This must be seen as one of the positive aspects of any screening programme, in that it adds a third course of action to the previously limited options of either continuing the pregnancy in the knowledge that the baby is not normal or terminating its life.

At the moment, the range of conditions that can be treated is small—but then ultrasound has only been widely available for just over a decade. On its own, the use of ultrasound technology would be of limited benefit, but it can become more powerful when combined with some of the miniature surgical instruments that are being invented for keyhole surgery.

Blood disorders

Rhesus incompatibility

Rhesus negative women need to discover the Rhesus group of their unborn babies early in pregnancy (see Rhesus factor in chapter 6). If the baby is found to be Rhesus positive and the mother is Rhesus negative, doctors will keep a regular check on the baby's ongoing growth. Any slow-down in growth indicates that the baby's blood is deteriorating. The only step now is to perform a blood transfusion, placing new Rhesus-positive blood into the baby.

To do this, a needle will be passed into the womb and on into one of the baby's blood vessels. There are two commonly used points of insertion, one in the umbilical cord, and one directly into a blood vessel in the baby's liver. This, of course, means pushing the needle into the baby, but it has the advantage that it is much less likely to damage the blood vessel than if the needle is pushed into the umbilical cord, and so reduces the chance of any permanent damage. After this procedure you will be asked to attend the clinic frequently for further monitoring, because the baby may need further transfusions of blood.

Each transfusion carries the risk of causing a miscarriage, so as soon as the baby has developed enough to survive well outside the womb, doctors are likely to recommend that they induce a slightly early delivery. Once the baby is out and detached from the mother, he or she will no longer receive the damaging antibodies and his or her blood will soon recover.

Congenital blood disorders

A few attempts have been made to treat unborn babies who have a rare disorder called severe combined immunodeficiency, and do not produce the white blood cells that fight disease. The problem is caused by a failure of the baby's bone marrow to manufacture these white cells and the condition is usually fatal by the age of two.

However, it seems that if the condition is diagnosed before the baby is 12–16 weeks of gestation, it might be possible to treat. A doctor working in Michigan, USA, pioneered an operation which involves three separate injections of healthy bone marrow into the baby's abdomen. The cells are taken up into the unborn baby's bloodstream and transported to the bones, where they appear to multiply and produce disease-fighting white blood cells.

This technique would fail in a child or adult unless the bone marrow matches, and identical donors are often hard to find. However, it appears that an unborn baby will not reject non-identical blood types at this stage of development, so the blood type doesn't need to be matched as precisely.

The technique is still considered to be experimental and other doctors say they have tried it and it doesn't work. However, it serves to point the way towards possible future treatments for thalassaemia or sickle-cell anaemia.

Kidneys and bladder

It is rare, but occasionally the tubes leading from the kidneys to the bladder are either missing or blocked, or the tube leading out from the bladder is similarly not functioning. Under ultrasound guidance, doctors can place small tubes called catheters in various places, which temporarily drain the accumulating fluid and allow normal development. This is only a stopgap operation and the root cause of the problem will need to be dealt with after birth.

Hydrocephalus

In this rare situation (1 in 1,000 births), fluid accumulates in the skull and prevents the brain developing properly, a condition called hydrocephalus. To prevent the damaging effects of this situation, a few operations have been performed in which a little tube has been inserted into the baby's head, allowing fluid around the brain to drain into the amniotic fluid. With the tube in place, the brain develops normally and then surgeons can sort out the drainage problem after the baby has been born.

However, the outcome from the first operations was so poor that most doctors believe that it is not ethical to continue with this form of surgery at the moment.

Diaphragmatic hernias

Within the body there are several sheets of muscle that divide up internal compartments. If one of these sheets tears, the contents of that compartment will spill out and cause trouble.

One of the largest such muscles is the diaphragm. This separates the abdomen, containing the stomach and intestines, from the thorax, which contains the heart and lungs. If it tears, some of the intestines spill into the thorax, thus putting pressure on the lungs. This prevents them from developing properly. The baby is therefore born with a very small lung capacity and will struggle to get enough oxygen. Soon after birth the baby will need an operation to close the hernia, giving the lungs the space they need to grow and work.

However, using ultrasound and microsurgery, a few surgeons have repaired the hernia before the baby is born, thus keeping the intestines in place and allowing the lungs to grow properly. At the moment, it is too early to know whether there is a real benefit from these operations.

Heart conditions

A few heroic attempts have been made to save the lives of unborn babies by operating on their hearts before they were born. In one operation, surgeons used a heated wire to burn a passage through the blocked valve to allow blood to flow into the artery leading to the lungs. The operation was conducted by passing the wire through the woman's abdominal wall, and into a vessel in the baby. The wire was then wriggled around into the baby's heart, where it could set to work.

Without the operation, the baby's heart and lungs would not have grown properly, leaving him in a very poor state at birth. With the operation successfully performed, the baby stood a much greater chance of survival, which was what happened. He did need further operations after being born but now lives a reasonably normal life.

The surgeons involved expressed cautious optimism that this sort of procedure could become routine. They point out that paediatricians are getting much better at looking after and curing sick children, so the need to solve problems before birth might be receding just as it becomes possible.

Future possibilities

Surgical teams based, for the most part, on the west coast of America have been performing partial Caesarean sections and operating on the unborn baby before returning the fetus to the warmth and safety of the womb. Such operations have so far had little success, in that a miscarriage often follows hard on the heels of the operation. However, while these operations can only be seen as experimental at the moment, the pace of change suggests that one day they may be more successful—who knows, they may even become commonplace.

While there is a distinct element of amazement and

sometimes revulsion at the idea of operating on an unborn baby, it has a number of positive elements. First, an unborn baby is plugged into the world's best life-support machine, in his own private, sterile pool. He is therefore in an ideal position to take it easy and recover gently from an operation. Secondly, scientists are realizing that any wounds inflicted on an unborn baby tend to heal without leaving a scar. This would be a great advantage if you needed to perform major abdominal or thoracic surgery, or operate to repair a cleft lip.

Epilogue

So the question is, what are you going to do? We've watched the developing baby grow and seen the developmental stages at which each test can be carried out. We've noted that many of the tests are screening tests and as such only indicated the relative risk of an individual being affected, rather than saying 'yes, the baby is healthy,' or 'no, there is some problem.' We've also seen that the tests used to diagnose more definitely the health status of an unborn baby carry with them a substantial risk of inducing a miscarriage.

The medical profession is united behind the idea that the person most influenced by the decision should be in control, and in this situation European law considers that person to be the mother. Along with the freedom to decide, this places the responsibility of any decision on her shoulders. She will hopefully be supported in this task by the baby's father, but antenatal tests push people into areas of science and ethics that they have never encountered before, facing questions like: When does a human being's life start? Where do the unborn baby's rights fit in? Do these rights change if tests show that he or she is not completely normal? But who, after all, is normal? Do the rights of the unborn child override the rights of existing family members—or do the rights of existing family members override those of the unborn child? How is the couple's own relationship going to be affected by the arrival of a child with a disability?

I hope the information in this book has gone some way to helping you make decisions that you are happy to live with. The best time to start thinking about the issues is before you embark on any tests—probably even better would be to start thinking about them before getting pregnant. Inevitably, many people will only start their research after they get a test result that indicates possible problems. Even the health professionals who spend every day working in the area find it difficult to give solid advice, because they are often unsure what they would do in a similar situation.

In researching for this book I was struck by two things. First, the similarity between current screening practice and eugenics. And secondly, the cost of screening programmes.

Eugenics literally means well born. The idea is that, one way or another, a society chooses to prevent people passing undesirable traits on to the next generation. Consequently, each generation should become healthier than the one before. The eugenic movement started in the USA around the end of the nineteenth century and the theme was picked up in Nazi Germany as Hitler sought to establish a pure race. Most people feel extremely uncomfortable with this period of recent history. After all, what right do we have to say that someone should not be allowed to have children, and what right do we have to select a range of conditions that we wish to eradicate?

I was therefore surprised to see how calmly many health professionals take the issue of screening for fetal abnormality, as very often this sets out to achieve similar goals—namely to remove certain types of abnormality and improve the genetic health of the population. Some have now started calmly using the term 'eugenic abortion' to refer to abortions for fetal abnormality. The recent history of eugenics should act as a warning signal and should make us look long and hard at our motivations for giving or having tests. Tests can have value if they give individuals choice and increased control over their lives, but there is danger in allowing this to progress into a mechanism for a national cleansing policy.

I was also surprised to discover how much we are prepared to spend to identify those unborn babies who have some disability. Estimating the cost of providing particular health programmes is very difficult. But one study indicated that the cost of the screening programme aimed at identifying babies with Down's syndrome was between £15,000 and £100,000 per affected baby that is detected.[1] Whatever the exact figure, it seems to be a lot of money in a health service that we are constantly being told is strapped for cash.

Some states in the USA now pick up the bill for amniocentesis and genetic counselling, rather than leaving it to the whim of the insurance companies. They do this not out of a sense of generosity, but because they hope that expectant parents will abort deformed fetuses rather than carry the babies to term. These states believe it is cheaper to fund the testing than to foot the bill for the care of these babies.

Antenatal testing is here to stay. It is driven by our desire to know that our offspring are healthy, but operates by identifying unborn babies that have some form of abnormality. My anxiety is mainly for couples for whom the tests identify an abnormality, and are suddenly launched into the ordeal of having to make massive decisions without any preparation. I also worry for the others who relax as the tests say the baby is probably OK, and are devastated when a problem is discovered at birth.

As far as antenatal testing is concerned, I think the bottom line is that everyone needs to consider what they want out of antenatal screening and then take the tests that can provide that information and avoid any others. At the same time they need to recognize the limitations of the tests. No tests can ever say that your baby is healthy; at best they can only rule out certain diseases.

Pete Moore

Notes

[1] Wald, N. & Watt, H., 'When marginal costs and benefits should be used in screening', British Medical Journal, 1996, 12: 1041–41.

Glossary

alpha-fetoprotein (AFP)

A protein made by the unborn baby that finds its way into the mother's bloodstream. The amount present in the mother's blood can indicate whether the baby has spina bifida or Down's syndrome. The AFP test is performed on a sample of the mother's blood taken from her arm.

amniocentesis

In this test, a sample of the baby's cells from the amniotic fluid is taken for laboratory analysis. The sample is taken by inserting a long syringe needle through the mother's amniotic wall into the amniotic sac. There is a 1 in 200 risk of miscarriage.

amniotic fluid

The fluid that surrounds the baby in the womb. It is made up largely of fetal urine and fluid that is produced in the baby's lungs, which flows out of the unborn baby's mouth.

antenatal

Before birth, or during pregnancy.

Bart's triple test

Also referred to as the triple test, the Bart's test and sometimes just as maternal serum screening. This measures three substances in the woman's blood—AFP, and two hormones (unconjugated oestriol and human chorionic gonadotrophin).

Braxton Hicks

Small contractions of the muscle of the womb. They occur late in pregnancy and help train the muscles for childbirth.

chromosomal abnormalities

Gross damage to the whole chromosomes.

Chorionic villus sampling (CVS)

A sample of the baby's cells is taken from the developing placenta. They are analysed in a laboratory.

congenital

Present at birth. Congenital diseases are ones that you are born with but have not necessarily inherited from either parent.

genetic abnormality

This is caused when there is a faulty single gene, inherited from parents.

lanugo hair

A fine hairy down which starts to grow in the fourth and fifth months of pregnancy and eventually covers the whole of the baby's body. However, during the ninth month of pregnancy it disappears in most cases, so you will usually only see it on premature babies.

neonatal

Newborn, normally a baby who is within a month of birth.

neural tube defects (NTDs)

A group of problems that originate in the first few weeks of pregnancy, resulting in either anencephaly, hydrocephalus or spina bifida.

nuchal scan

An early ultrasound scan that measures the thickness of folds at the back of the baby's neck. If the fold is wider than normal, it may indicate that the baby has Down's syndrome.

mosaicism

A situation where a genetic abnormality does not occur in all of the cells in the person's body.

Maternal serum alpha-fetoprotein (MSAFP)

Another name for AFP—*see above.*

penetrance

The extent to which a person is affected by a genetic disease.

pre-eclampsia

A serious disorder affecting up to 7 per cent of pregnancies. It is characterized by high blood pressure (hypertension), tissue swelling (oedema) and protein in the woman's urine (proteinuria). It can be accompanied by headaches, vomiting, abdominal pain and visual disturbances and may develop in the second half of pregnancy. If severe and/or left untreated, the condition can cause the death of the baby and/or the woman.

prenatal

Before birth, or during pregnancy.

pregnancy toxaemia

Sometimes used as another term for pre-eclampsia.

quadruple test

Also known as Bart's quad test, this is a test which measures the three substances that the Bart's triple test measures, plus an additional type of human chorionic hormone.

ultrasound scan

Considered the least harmful pregnancy test. An image of the baby is projected onto a screen.

vernix

A creamy, greasy substance which covers the unborn baby's skin and protects it from the effects of being constantly bathed in fluid.

Support agencies

Antenatal Screening Service
The Wolfson Institute
St Bartholomew's and the Royal London School of Medicine
 and Dentistry
Charterhouse Square
London EC1M 6BQ
Tel: 0171 982 6293/4

Association for Spina Bifida and Hydrocephalus
ASBAH House
42 Park Road
Peterborough
Cambridgeshire PE1 3UQ
Tel: 01733 555988

British Tay-Sachs Foundation
Jewish Care
221 Golders Green Road
London NW11 9DQ
Tel: 0181 458 3282

CARE for Life
53 Romney Street
London SW1P 3RF
Tel: 0171 233 0455
*A Christian charity that provides advice and support for couples facing
decisions about caring for unborn babies.*

CLAPA
Cleft Lip and Palate Association
1 Eastwood Gardens
Kenton
Newcastle NE3 3DQ
Tel: 0191 285 9396

CRUSE
Cruse House
126 Sheen Road
Richmond
Surrey TW9 1UR
Tel: 0181 940 4818
The national organization for the widowed and their children.

Contact-a-family
170 Tottenham Court Road
London W1P 0HA
Tel: 0171 383 3555
*Provides information and brings together families who have children with
similar problems.*

Cystic Fibrosis Trust
Alexandra House
Bromley Road
Bromley
Kent BR1 3RS
Tel: 0181 464 7211

Down's Syndrome Association
155 Mitcham Road
London SW17 9PG
Tel: 0181 682 4001

Down's Syndrome Screening Service
Institute of Epidemiology
34 Hyde Terrace
Leeds LS2 9LN
Tel: 0113 233 6770

Haemophilia Society
123 Westminster Bridge Road
London SE1 7HR
Tel: 0171 928 2020

National AIDS Helpline
Tel: 0800 567123

National Society for PKU(Phenylketonuria)
7 Southfield Close
Willen
Milton Keynes
Buckinghamshire MK12 9LL
Tel: 01908 691653

RELATE
Herbert Gray College
Little Church Street
Rugby
Warwickshire CV21 3AP
Tel: 01788 573241
Provides marriage guidance for couples whose marriage is under threat.

SATFA (Support Around Termination for Fetal Abnormality)
73 Charlotte Street
London W1P 1LB
Tel: 0171 631 0285

Sickle Cell Society
54 Station Road
London NW10 4UA
Tel: 0181 961 7795/8346

UK Thalassaemia Society
107 Nightingale Lane
London N8 7QY
Tel: 0181 348 0437

Ask your local Paediatric Development Unit or health visitor for information about local support groups.

Further reading

Rosemary Dodds, *The Stress of Tests in Pregnancy* (National Childbirth Trust, February 1997). Summary of a National Childbirth Trust antenatal screening survey.

Barbara Katz Rothman, *The Tentative Pregnancy* (Pandora Press, London, 1986). A discussion of the effect that antenatal screening has had on pregnancy.

Brendan McCarthy, *Fertility and Faith* (Inter Varsity Press, Leicester, 1997). Contains a thorough review of biblical texts relating to the status of the human embryo and fetus.

Pete Moore, *Trying for a Baby* (Lion Publishing, Oxford, 1996). Contains a discussion of the moral status of an unborn baby.

Lennart Nilsson, *A Child is Born* (New Edition—Transworld Publishers, London, 1990). A full-colour version of his remarkable collection of photographs, charting human development from conception to birth.

Index